THE YOGA OF KNOWLEDGE

The Yoga of Knowledge gives the necessary background to pursue one's quest in whatever direction chosen with the maximum benefit. The Yoga of Knowledge embraces all that can be known, and helps one to realise—not necessarily in the mental way—all that is still unknown.

Most of the presentations in this book are followed by questions and answers touching a wide range of topics not necessarily related to the theme of the talks but of considerable spiritual importance.

THE YOGA OF KNOWLEDGE

Based on Sri Aurobindo's Synthesis of Yoga

M.P. Pandit

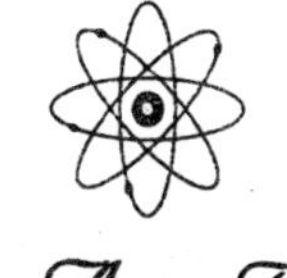

New Age Books

ISBN: 81-7822-078-4

First Indian Edition: 2002

Second Edition: USA, 1986

Published by arrangement with
Lotus Press, USA

Published by
NEW AGE BOOKS
A-44 Naraina Phase I
New Delhi-110 028 (INDIA)
Email: nab@vsnl.in
Website: www.newagebooksindia.com

For Sale in South Asia Only

Printed in India
at Shri Jainendra Press
A-45 Naraina Phase-I New Delhi-110 028

Contents:

PREFACE

This series of talks based on *The Synthesis of Yoga* of Sri Aurobindo was given at the Centre, Peace, Auroville (1972—1973). The first volume, already issued, comprises the talks on *The Yoga of Works.* The present one, the second, covers *The Yoga of Knowledge.* Most of the presentations are followed by questions and answers touching a wide range of topics not necessarily related to the theme of the talks but of considerable spiritual importance.

1

The Object of Knowledge

It is understood that in an integral path there are no rigid distinctions: a separate yoga of works, a distinct yoga of knowledge, and quite a different yoga of love. All three are lines of effort. Each individual starts on that line which is most congenial to him, but he knows and he takes steps to combine all the three. The other two may be woven around the central line chosen, but each one extends into the other.

In this discipline, the yoga of knowledge occupies a very important place. Even though one may not make it his principal concern, it is necessary to know at least in outline the principles and truths expounded in the yoga of knowledge. I may be a sincere and dedicated worker, my line of evolution having prepared me for the manifestation of the Divine in the way of the movement of will. Still, there is a difference between one who does works without being conscious of the full bearings and one who knows the background, the process, and the goal of the path that he is treading.

The yoga of knowledge gives the necessary background to pursue one's quest in whatever direction chosen with the maximum benefit. When I work, for instance, I must know what it is that works. Is it my body or my vital energy, and what place has my mind in it? It is easy to say, "Surrender your works, don't desire the fruit of works", but what exactly is the transmutation that takes place in one's being and consciousness? I may read something in a book, I may be told something by my senior, and make a resolve. But how exactly is it to be translated, how effected by the various faculties of my being? And what are the different faculties that are patent or latent in the human system? What relation have they to the quest of the soul? These and other elements of the requisite knowledge are given in the yoga of knowledge.

Similarly, if my choice is the way of love, if it is natural and spontaneous for me to feel the flow of devotion and love for the Divine, if I feel carried away in a flood of oneness, a feeling of harmony, without my effort, can I just let myself sail in that current? Is there no danger of the ego, of the unpurified vital being assuming control at some stage and convincing me that I have realised the Divine as Bliss? To guard myself from that eventuality, I must know from where the emotions rise, what is the difference between human emotions and divine love, between a mental conception of oneness and the soul's experience of oneness, between a mental construction of unity and a spontaneous flow of oneness? From where do they arise? How do they work? All this again presupposes a minimum knowledge of my psychological being.

But I do not live alone. However indrawn I may be, withdrawn from the world, I breathe at every moment the air of those around me. Known or unknown to me, ideas, thoughts, emotions, perceptions and conceptions impinge upon me from all sides. I may delude myself into the belief that I am the author, the originator of all these movements, but the facts are otherwise. I should know which movements are my own, which come upon me from others, and which arise from universal nature, not through anyone in particular. For this again, I must know the arrangement of the cosmic orders of existence — the several planes of existence that constitute the universe, that transcend this world — and how exactly they are related to the various parts of my being. If I am the microcosm, in what precise manner am I related to the macrocosm? Unless I know the exact correspondences and the points of contact between my being and the universal being, I will not be in a position to stop unwanted incursions or to project from my soul such movements as I would be moved to direct towards others. This too requires a knowledge of the constitution of the universe.

From where has this universe originated? Has it just accidentally come to be? Is it that God one day felt the impulse and said, "Let there be creation", and the creation came to be? Or is there a process? If so, is that process initiated by a whim or is there an ordered conception, a law of truth, behind it? And what exactly is the nature of this truth? Is this truth what is meant by truth in our manuals of ethics? Or is it something dynamic that impels the evolution of the universe and all that constitutes the universe?

All these topics, all these items of knowledge which one must know — whether in detail or in substance — are dealt with in the yoga of knowledge. The yoga of knowledge that Sri Aurobindo expounds embraces all that can be known, and helps one to realise — not necessarily in the mental way — all that is still unknown.

In this respect, the yoga of knowledge that we are going to study is different from the traditional yoga of knowledge. At any rate in the East, the path of knowledge, *jnanayoga*, has come to mean and has been systematized in such a way that the unfoldment of the yoga of knowledge depends upon one's withdrawal — the withdrawal of the knower from the world, from the universe. Here, the knowledge of the constitution of the world and the universe is not very relevant. This traditional yoga of knowledge has for its object the Supreme — a reality, an absolute which it conceives to be transcendent, to reach which one has to reject the world which acts as a veil, a barrier, a mould of imprisonment. By whatever means, this world of ignorance, this formation of falsehood has to be rejected. As one rejects and detaches oneself from the objective world, one opens the doors to the subjective. One turns in the direction of the Self which is alone, austere, unconnected, aloof. There are lines of the yoga of knowledge which perceive the reality above the universe, wholly transcendent, absolutely unconcerned, "without sinews", "without scars", "without imperfections", in its grand aloofness. It is unknowable — the mind and the senses fall back from it in their attempt to reach it. But it can be realised in the being; for that, everything has to fall silent — then one gets a glimpse of the reality.

This is the fundamental assumption on which the traditional yoga of knowledge proceeds. The method is one of discrimination between the true and the false — what I consider to be true and false — the transient and the eternal, the temporary and the permanent, spirit and matter. There has to be an incessant action of discrimination at every level of life, followed by the rejection — first detachment, and then rejection — of what is not true, what is not relevant or pertinent. This way of discrimination and detachment is the principal method of the traditional yoga of knowledge.

You have heard of Shankara, the great philosopher and yogin whom Sri Aurobindo describes as perhaps the greatest intellect that ever lived on earth. He has come to occupy an extraordinarily predominant position in the philosophical and spiritual thought of India. It was he who completed the circle of negation started by Buddha. Buddha did not say that the world is false, all that he said was, "The world is a place of suffering; one has to find a way out of it." Shankara said, "Whether it is a world of suffering or joy, pleasure or pain, it is a world of ignorance and falsehood, it has no substantial reality; it is to be rejected." The philosophy he propounded is known as *advaita*, monism, which posits only one reality — the Brahman as he called it — which is aloof, on the bosom of which an inscrutable power called *maya* plays and directs the fantasy of worlds after worlds. Man has in him, he said, a Self which is a reflection or a spark of that reality. If only man would withdraw his association with the formations of ignorance, he would realise his true nature and become one with the Brahman.

Shankara's whole philosophy has been epitomised in a celebrated hymn called "The Hymn of Nirvana", ascribed to him. Rendered in English, this is the substance of the hymn:

> I am not the mind, not the intellect, not the ego, not the stuff of consciousness. I am not the ear, not the tongue, neither the nose nor the eyes. I am not the ether, not the earth, not fire, not wind, but of the form, of the consciousness that is Bliss. I am pure Shiva, I am Shiva.
>
> I am not life-force, I am not the fivefold movement of breath, not the seven elements, nor am I the five sheaths. Not speech, not hands, not feet, not any other sense organ, but I am the consciousness that is Bliss, the pure Shiva.
>
> I am neither attraction nor repulsion, neither greed nor delusion belong to me, no intoxication of power, no jealousy. Neither have I religion, nor any object to be fulfilled, no desire — not even liberation. I am pure consciousness, pure Shiva, pure being.
>
> Neither merit nor demerit, neither friendship, neither happiness nor unhappiness, no ritual of mantra or holy places, no Vedas, no sacrifices. Neither am I food nor the eating of food nor the enjoyer of food. I am pure consciousness, pure being.
>
> Not death, not doubt, nor sense of class, neither father nor mother nor birth are mine. I have no friends, no relations, there is neither teacher nor disciple for me. I am pure consciousness, pure being.
>
> I am thoughtless, no thought moves in me. There is no form in my consciousness because all my senses are spread everywhere, they are not confined to my body. I am not attached; for one

> who is not attached, where is the question of liberation? Nobody can measure me, I am measureless. I am pure consciousness, pure bliss.

This "Hymn of Nirvana" illustrates and sums up the way and the aim of the traditional yoga of knowledge.

You would have felt or perceived that this expression doesn't come from the mind. It proceeds out of the fullness of a great experience, a capital realisation, without which, Sri Aurobindo points out, the mind cannot be entirely free. The experience upon which the hymn is based proceeds from a deep level of spiritual certitude, when one is freed from the bonds that hold one down and is identified with the reality in its aspects of absolute peace — aloof, alone, beyond. One has to realise this aspect of the reality as a crown of one's labours of disassociation and detachment from the movements and formulations of lower nature.

But that is not all. The traditional way stops at this experience. It is an overwhelming experience, which one meets on the borders of the mind as it crosses into the regions of the spiritual mind. One is simply knocked over by the solidity of this peace that depends upon nothing, of this rock of silence that cannot be moved by any number of violent revolutions of the mind or vital. It is overpowering. If one chooses to stop there, one shortens one's horizons, one stops short of one's fuller destiny.

Sri Aurobindo notes that he himself had this experience a number of times — when he was in politics, when he was touring. But he had a perception that that was not the whole truth. It was revealed to him, as it is revealed to all who have that experience and who have the patience to wait, that it is only a foundation, a standing ground for emerging into the greater glories of the Spirit. Unless one arrives at this solid foundation of peace, of release, of an essential identity with the Divine, one cannot support the revelation of the glories of

Power, Knowledge, and Bliss that await one on the heights of the being, that wait to be first embodied and then manifested.

The battle is not won by a release from the lower nature. This is only the beginning of the second step. The yoga of knowledge as enunciated by Sri Aurobindo shows precisely how man has to pass through these capital experiences, take their strength, and equip himself to receive the much that is still unmanifested. There are enough hints in the ancient scriptures that though many who are liberated may go beyond, there are some great ones who remain to do the great work — the work of reaching the joys of heaven to all beings on earth, of functioning as vehicles for the transmission of the divine consciousness and energies to earth, of being instruments for effecting the transformation of life, converting the earth into a kingdom of God.

If one is not satisfied with taking a leap straight from the spiritual heights of the mind to the absolute Transcendent, if one does not close one's eyes to the tiers, the gradations of existence that open before one as one ascends the stair of existence, there is much that waits to be done. It is the special distinction of this teaching that more stress is laid on manifestation, on working out the concealed glories of God on earth, than on liberating man from the earth into a beyond from which he never returns. For surely that is not the aim or the end for which nature has laboured milleniums. Man has a glorious destiny, but also a noble task awaiting him. He has to be a doer of works, he has to perceive that as much as he is real, the world also is real. The way of knowledge points out, step by step, that the reality of life on earth is not exhausted by its material appearance. The physical is not all; the brain and the nerves are not all. There is some vibrant power that makes them living. It shows next that even this life-power which energises matter, which energises everything that would otherwise remain dead, is not the sole explanation. When we analyse the life energies we come across rudiments of mind, workings of a consciousness, and we stumble on to the third truth — the formulation of mind as a principle. But even the mind is not a self-sufficing explanation; the mind itself points to a truth beyond it.

In this way — by a progressive analysis of the different grades of existence, without and within — man the knower, the follower of the yoga of knowledge comes to perceive that there is one mighty Consciousness which formulates and organises itself in different configurations, appearances, and vibrations at different levels. And it simply will not do to confine ourselves to just one or two or three layers and close our eyes to the larger levels of existence that are beyond. All have to be realised — the reality of the whole of life from matter to the highest spirit. The reality is to be experienced, embodied and manifested. This then is the object of our pursuit of knowledge.

Any questions?

Would you say that rajayoga is part of the yoga of knowledge?

Rajayoga can be one of the means for pursuing the yoga of knowledge. Particularly the mechanical side of it can help in the gathering of the mental faculties, subjecting them to a certain process of purification, centralising them around the truth that you want to realise, and in separating the soul from nature. In this way, rajayoga can be of help. It can help in our yoga, it can help in any yoga, but certain parts of it like *pranayama* are unsafe unless pursued under the eye of a teacher who can guide. And it is not part of rajayoga to have the soul master nature; the soul detaches itself from nature. This yoga attempts or aims, once the detachment is effected, to acquire mastery over nature so that what is *prakriti*, what is ignorant nature, is converted into *shakti*, into the self-power of the divinity within.

2

The Status of Knowledge and the Purified Understanding

We have discussed what is the object of our knowledge, the goal that we intend to reach by following the way of knowledge. At the end of our last discussion we were in the presence of the divine reality that ensouls all forms and movements; the eternal, on the bosom of which all moves in time; the immutable, on which all spatial formations move. We visualised the Self, which is the substratum of all forms in creation. We posited an omnipresent reality as the object of our knowledge. And what is the means to reach this object, the precise line of knowledge that we are to pursue?

When we speak of knowledge, normally we mean the knowledge picked up by our outgoing senses — touching their objects, reporting back to the mind — and the mind's rendering of that data into terms of the intellect. But this process of knowledge, sense knowledge, touches only the surfaces of things, the externals on which the senses impinge and report back. It does not go beyond the appearances; and as a consequence, we are obliged to revise the knowledge so arrived at as we touch, in the course of life, different and deeper levels of existence.

What appears to be true on the surface is no longer true when we probe a little deeper. That is why the Mother calls the senses liars. Whether the senses grasp things as they are, even on the surface, is doubtful. Doubtful because each sense operation of the individual is directed by a motive, whether he is conscious of it or not. The motive of desire, the motive of ego, the motive of thought — each wants knowledge to be in a particular bent, and the senses consciously or unconsciously obey that impulse and grasp things accordingly. The knowledge of the senses is a biased knowledge. Obviously this knowledge is unsatisfactory in the quest in which we are engaged.

Even the knowledge that is of a higher type than sense knowledge, the knowledge that is obtained by mental interpretation of the data brought by the senses, is doubtful. The mind interprets in a particular way. The same data presented to five different minds would be interpreted in five different ways. The mind is interested in understanding things in a particular way. It is too interested, desirous, to be an objective interpreter of knowledge through the data supplied to it.

One may ask, in that case, whether all the knowledge on which we act is useless. Certainly not. The old Upanishads make a distinction between the higher knowledge and the lower knowledge. It is recorded in a three or four thousand year old text that when Narada, the famous sage — who had undergone several austerities and had gone to the end of the knowledge that could be garnered through a study of science and art — realised that he had known only verbal knowledge and not the truth of things, he invoked the Divine as the Son of God, the Eternal Boy, Sanatkumara, and appealed to him: "I have studied the sixty-four arts and sciences that are sanctified in the name of God. But at the end of it all, I have realised that I know nothing. I know only words, and what the words say. I am not in the presence of the knowledge that is living."

And it is recorded that the grace, in the form of Sanatkumara, took compassion and answered his prayer to show him the other shore beyond the darkness of Ignorance. There he speaks of the lower knowledge and the higher knowledge; the lower knowledge consists of the various branches of learning, arts and sciences. He says, "They do not help to reach the Self. It is only the higher knowledge which takes you beyond the forms and appearances, which puts you in the proximity of the one Self, the Eternal, where knowledge is attained by means other than the mental. That is the higher and the true knowledge." But the Upanishad takes care to record that the lower knowledge is a necessary step to the higher one.

These lower branches of learning — knowledge based upon the data of the senses and built up by the intellect — give us the truth of the processes, at any rate certain processes, in creation, the processes of nature. Perhaps we are not yet in possession of the processes of higher nature, but the intricate workings of the machinery of the lower nature, earth nature, have been exposed and made familiar to our minds. To this extent that knowledge has served humanity, and we record our gratitude to modern science and the older sciences for the service that they have rendered in familiarising man with the processes, the operations of truth.

But when we want to know the truth of things — not just the process by which it works — and why it works in a particular way, we are in another realm of consciousness. And to enter this realm, to understand its mysteries, we need to cultivate other means of knowledge. Sense knowledge and intellectual knowledge are to be left behind once their purpose of sharpening and preparing the mind is served.

Even the highest processes and means of the traditional Indian yoga of knowledge, deliberation and discrimination, do not give us the truth of things. A traditional *jnanayogin*, a practitioner of the Vedantic yoga of knowledge, takes, during his meditation or concentration or communion with God, each form that comes before him and deliberates upon it — what is its nature? why and how does it come into being? — discriminates its elements of the temporal from the eternal, the true from the false, and rejects the untrue and temporal. This successive deliberation and discrimination is practised by him till all that belongs to this temporal and transitory world is shut from his consciousness.

But in this yoga, the highest purpose served by deliberation and discrimination is that of removing the cobwebs of ignorance, darkness, and obscurity, removing the obstructions. Their role is to purify, negatively, but there it ends. We have to build upon the ground cleared by this twin operation of deliberation and discrimination. After its full working, after it has rejected the impressions heaped up by the senses and analysed and collated by the intellect in its own way, there comes another operation, the spiritual operation of vision.

One may have read, heard from others, intellectualised, and formed a certain definite idea of what the reality is, of what the Self is. I may say, and my mind may be convinced, that the reality is one, immutable, and eternal. But there it stops. It is a mental idea or knowledge which does not have a concrete impact on the rest of my being. Does it change my movements in life? Does it really affect my attitude to men and things? How far does an intellectual conviction carry man? What the mind is convinced of, the intellect has built at its level. It can have its full power only when one has the direct vision of the reality. It is just as on the physical plane where we may hear of many things and form ideas — from books, reports, imagination — but only get the full impact when the thing is presented to our physical vision. Then we form a direct contact and the thing becomes part of us. Thereafter, for the rest of our lives, it remains with us. Similarly, on the subtler spiritual plane, the knowledge has not yet become real unless one has or is vouchsafed the vision of the reality, the Divine as light; a representation, a direct ray of light of the Divine falls on one and makes a concrete impact.

But even this vision of light or form is only the first touch. The eye that sees is not the entire being. Man consists of so many parts, and each part has to realise its truth in the Self. The Self projects itself in the form of the mind, the heart, the life-force, even of the body. Each formation, each formulation has got to go back to its indwelling, inherent Self and realise that truth. The mind has to realise the direct sense of its knowledge of the supreme reality — say for instance as existence, consciousness, and bliss. The heart has to go back and realise the truth of love — that it is not the changing human emotion that we call love, but the unchanging, independent truth of a love that pours itself on all, irrespective of their reactions or recognitions. Similarly the life-force has to realise its truth in the Self as a projection of the consciousness-force of the Divine. Even the physical learns — in the course of *tapasya*, spiritual discipline — that it is not a veil, but it is an embodiment of the physical Self. Thus the revelation that started with the vision has to be built up and established at each level of the being; vision followed by experience. Experience gives us a touch of the reality.

But that is not the end. So many spiritual careers have come to an untimely end simply because one experience was taken to be the total realisation. An experience is one point of contact. Each one has to be confirmed repeatedly, organised, established in the being, and built into a realisation. Experience is the seed out of which the fruit of realisation is to emerge. And when this experience of the reality is repeatedly confirmed by evocation and opening oneself, when it is organised in the rest of the being, then comes the stage of identity with the Divine. When there is identity there is no separate knower, one becomes one with the known. The trinity of the knower, the known, and the knowledge fuses into one. There is a complete realisation of the reality.

This passage from the human level to the Divine, however, is long. It has to proceed through many stages. But largely this process is twofold: the part which constitutes purification of the members of our being and, as a consequence, the part that constitutes the illumination of the being by the higher consciousness towards which we move. Unless each part of ourselves — or to begin with, the leading part — is purified of the dross of the lower nature, of its ignorance, remnants of falsehood and egoism, unless the part that leads and thereafter the parts that follow are subjected to a radical process of purification, it is idle to expect progress to be made.

As purification proceeds, the higher consciousness responds by sending forth its rays of light, peace, and joy to strengthen the members that are being purified. Thus there is no clear demarcation between the two processes of purification and illumination. They go side by side. As purification proceeds, there is a larger opening effected where the illumining rays of the higher consciousness are received. And as the rays act upon the levels that are cleared, the area is extended and resistances in related regions break down so that more parts become purified.

In man, the part which leads — particularly in the yoga of knowledge that we are at present considering — is understanding. It is imperative, then, that the understanding be purified. Unless it is, one is very likely to be much confused, to be misled; even with all good intentions one can be misled. Sri Aurobindo has written in a letter entitled "The Intermediate Zone", published in *The Riddle of this World*, a description of the hundred ways in which the mind can be dazzled, the understanding confused, and one can get completely lost in a zone of dazzling splendours, pleasing falsehoods. So, the understanding has to be purified.

Why else does the understanding need to be purified? As we have discussed, the mind itself, which is our instrument of knowledge, consists broadly of three layers. First, that with which an average man starts is the sense mind, the mind based upon the senses, which is full of impurities, unreliable evidences. Second, that part of the intellect which bases itself entirely on the reports of the sense mind — it interprets them, it builds knowledge based upon evident sense information. Third, what is called the reason proper, which analyses with cold logic and pretends to give complete, foolproof knowledge. But we know that though reason is a very good understudy, it is never a reliable master. Reason can support or contradict any proposition, it depends upon what we want it to do. And here is the danger: no operation of the human intellect, the thinking mind, is free from mixture, the interference of desire. Sri Aurobindo has written page after page describing how the undercurrent of desire inclines the reason, the logical mind to interpret and understand things in a particular way to suit the fulfillment of desire.

That desire, again, need not be the vital kind of desire for vital fulfillment; it can very well be a mental desire, a spiritual desire. To arrive at ideas and notions which we want or are fond of, to extol and exaggerate certain realisations which are dear to us — and to deprecate others — is the manifold desire that twists the operations of the intellect at its very source. What Sri Aurobindo calls "the impurity of will" — the will involved in an interested operation — contributes to the defective and faulty working of the understanding. Second, by habit the process has been built up of feeding the understanding from the sense level. That again brings another level of impurity. Third, there is, as just mentioned, the element of impurity in thought itself. We have, each one of us, pet ideas and notions; we want truth to be a particular way, want it to present itself in this manner or that form. This prejudges the issue, and the understanding is weighted in favour of our recognised or unrecognised notions and preferences.

These are the three impurities that are to be eliminated from our understanding. It is only then, Sri Aurobindo points out, that understanding comes into its own: it ceases to be an understanding and becomes an "overstanding" — standing above the movements and observing the truth in and behind them.

When the understanding is so purified and rectified, it is to be subjected to a twofold passivity. It recognises that the true knowledge is not to come from outside, but from within and from the heights of the being, behind and above. The understanding realises that there are levels of knowledge waiting to be tapped which pour themselves through intuition and revelation. All knowledge required — the knowledge of all that goes on, has gone on, and is to go on — is preserved at a level where what is called "the memory of the future" is stored. If the prepared understanding falls silent and awaits this revelation with a vigilance and a keenness, the contents pour themselves. But that too is not the end.

So, the formulations of the reality in terms of knowledge are poured into the upturned understanding that is purified. There is more. When in this process of purifying the understanding the thought mind is silenced, when it is shorn of disturbing mechanical thought-movements and just falls silent and nothing moves — like the waters of a lake as described by Patanjali, the ancient systematiser of yoga — then the reality reflects itself in its pure form. In silence one hears the Silence — one can hear the Silence — in peace the understanding dawns.

Any questions?

How does the manifestation as well as the realisation of the reality relate to time and space?

The supreme reality is above time and space. It is unchanging, immutable; you can't describe it as this or that. It is there. It is the manifestation of that truth that proceeds in terms of time and space. Even time and space are its own formulations. Time is the eternal as duration, space the infinite as extension. Now, it is this manifestation of the reality that is dynamic, changing, bringing forth new contents from the bosom of reality — moment to moment, age to age. And it is these truths, these aspects of the reality that reveal themselves, that are realised by man. There is no end to the aspects of the divine reality that can be realised by man.

But, on that account, there is no comparison in terms of superiority or inferiority, limited or unlimited. Each spiritual realisation, each realisation of one aspect of the reality, is valid, supremely valid.

The manifestation goes on. But the highest reality available to human consciousness at a given moment in time is called the supreme attainable reality. In the ancient Indian tradition, the highest attainable level of the reality was called Shiva, Brahman. But they were careful to posit that beyond that there is something about which we can neither say what it is nor what it is not. And, realise? realise what? When you come to the realisable summit you become one with it. There is nothing or no one further to realise thereafter.

Each avatar comes to realise and embody in human form and to make available to humanity a particular grade of truth, a particular potential of truth which is necessary at that stage in evolution. Necessarily, in terms of time, each successive avatar brings a fuller truth, in keeping with the more advanced stage of evolution of humanity. Sri Aurobindo has arrived at a time when humanity is ready for a more synthetic, rounded realisation of the reality than was possible before. All the realisations brought down and manifested by the great spiritual figures have been so many contributions leading to this fulfillment of the present age. Nobody ever said that this is the final realisation. Sri Aurobindo himself said that once you attain the supramental realisation and house the supramental consciousness, there are still further vistas. New avatars may come — though we may not call them avatars at that time — new manifestations will come; the vistas of the infinite are endless. There is no limit. We can't say this is the highest and no further. We are concerned only with what is the highest possible now for human consciousness. The rest is academic.

What is the place of the psychic guidance in this path of knowledge?

This is very interesting. Almost precisely the same question was put to me this morning. Somebody noted that I have said in one of my writings that one must refer each movement in day to day life to the psychic within, and asked how it is to be done. The question now is: what role does the psychic play in the practice of deliberation and discrimination aimed at purifying one's understanding? Where does the guidance of Sri Aurobindo and Mother come in?

Done purely as a mental operation, this process of deliberation and discrimination is a laborious one. It is called *vichara marga*, the way of enquiry, of mental scrutiny, in the Indian tradition. Very laborious. People spend hours analysing whether something is true or not. They lose themselves in rounds of speculation. It becomes a very dry endeavour, and the mind is apt to become a prisoner of the process that is intended to liberate it.

To prevent deliberation and discrimination from becoming a laborious and self-defeating project, one has to call in the aid of the psychic. After all, what is the psychic? The psychic centre is the point where the divine presence in each person stations itself. Whether you are aware of it or not, the presence is there. One has to first have the faith that it is there in the core of the heart. One doesn't have that knowledge immediately when starting on the path, so one has to take the word of those who have gone before. Having that faith, one must, in moments of meditation, concentration, or prayer, have an aspiration and call the Divine there to reveal itself. Exert that pressure on the Divine intensely during periods of meditation and, in a general way, have that remembrance and aspiration that it should reveal itself during the rest of the time.

If one has a sincere desire to have that presence manifest in oneself, gradually an awareness develops of something that is behind all this movement, separate, uninvolved. One has to fix one's consciousness there. Having found the point, thereafter by dwelling upon and paying attention to it, one has to extend its area. Gradually there is an articulate response to the aspiration. We need not now go into the further processes. Till that happens and also once it does, every time there is a contact with someone or some movement — whether sought for or it just impinges itself upon one — before reacting, one must step back and remember. There is no need to call it to guide; it is enough to remember the Divine within, and one will be guided. Similarly, whenever one is about to act, remember, and the centre of reference will develop. The centre of reference in one's life moves from the external mind to the soul, to the psychic. This is the idea.

But most of us here are so favourably circumstanced that we do not need to imagine or to conceive of the Divine or the psychic in the abstract. We have the Mother, who links us with the reality within ourselves and others, outside, everywhere. She embodies the divinity for us. Remember Mother everytime you act or react. This slowly yet dynamically builds up the Mother's consciousness in you, step by step, and it becomes a force. As her consciousness develops from being merely a centre of reference, the charge of the sadhana is eventually taken from your hands. Deliberation and discrimination will proceed spontaneously from that consciousness.

Sri Aurobindo and the Mother are dynamic presences in action in each one of us. One has only to remember and evoke the presence, and the guidance is there. After evoking the guidance, to follow it is our part; and it is there that most fail.

Sincerity, purity, receptivity — these are demanded.

When one knows that this is the true thing, yet one still persists, for any reason, in doing a different thing, the guidance will not repeat itself more than two or three times. Sincerity is the first step; then receptivity; then vigilance. When the guidance comes one has to act upon it without question.

The Divine helps even if one is weak and fails?

Certainly. Actually, as the Mother says, if you take one step, the Divine takes two. It may withdraw, but it doesn't leave, it waits. The moment you realise that you have made a mistake, that is enough, it comes. It gives you another chance, in fact many chances. Even the slightest realisation that you have not followed the guidance is enough. That is an implicit admission and a readiness to correct yourself. If you do not follow the guidance by sheer weakness and you know that you are at fault and repent, then you are still within the realm of the action of the grace. If you act out of ignorance or weakness, there is hope for redemption. The grace is there. Even for one who rejects the guidance, the grace acts, but in a different way. It acts through the operation, the compulsions of karma.

What is the relation between moral and psychic guidance?

Usually the ethical or moral guidance, the traditional injunctions, are sediments left in the mental and vital levels of an inherited past active in the present in which we live.

But the psychic is deeper. When the psychic guidance comes, there is a feeling of conviction. It doesn't admit of any question; it is transparent. It does not impose itself, it does not compel one to obey, but there it is, it shows itself. There is about it an atmosphere of certainty, a soft peace, a velvety background. If we do not accept the guidance it just retires. It does not demand that one obey it, though it carries a conviction about it.

One has to be silent. If one is not satisfied, one may mentally analyse whether it comes from the spiritual depths or from one's own understanding of what is right, ethical, or moral. If one is sincere and submits the problem to the Divine within or above, and just waits for a moment without struggling to get the reply, one does receive it. Mother says that because people are restless and want the answer immediately, they get their own answer. One has to wait in trust. At times it is good to forget about it for a while after submitting the problem. When one least expects it, it sails into the being, into the mind. The will of the mind has to be removed. One has to submit trustfully and wait.

One may say that a busy man in the street does not have the time to do all this, but this operation is not expected of him. It is expected of a seeker, and the seeker has the time. A person in the world who is a seeker within, has time within.

What about visions in receiving guidance?

Usually these visions or revelations in form — either in the form of light or of particular figures — do not come by our effort. They just reveal themselves when the consciousness is ready to receive them.

Now to make the consciousness ready, receptive, to bring it into a fit condition in which it can receive the impact, all the methods of concentration, a gathering meditation, a movement of rising prayer, a silent lapse of the consciousness, are used. These are means by which the condition is prepared for the revelation to take place. By whatever method, the outspread consciousness has to be gathered and presented.

This can even happen involuntarily in certain cases. Say in a moment of crisis or emergency, suddenly all the outer coverings fall away and the inner consciousness gathers without our effort. These are moments that the Divine waits for to reveal itself.

It can happen when one least expects it; the soul pushes forward. One may be in any circumstance and receive the vision; not a mental but a spiritual vision. A moment has arrived for the soul in its inner evolution — which goes on irrespective of what one does or does not do — to take a leap. All the outer senses are dulled and the inner ones come forward and take cognisance; though one may think that one has heard or seen with the physical senses.

So these are among the various possibilities open to man. But a seeker has to make the effort on his side to keep himself in a constant state of readiness for any revelation that may be shown to him, for any word that may reach him through anyone, or through none.

3

Concentration

Side by side with purification comes concentration. Sri Aurobindo describes purification and concentration as the feminine and masculine aspects of the process of yoga. Purification without concentration tends to remain a mere quietude. It is only if purification is backed up by and made use of by the process of concentration that it yields its full results. Most of the impurity in an individual is due to the fact that there is no willed concentration of the faculties of the mind or heart.

Man stands exposed to whatever impacts come upon him in the world, and it is only his surface mind that picks up a few contacts and establishes some sort of connection, a working relation, between them. The contacts are unregulated, and the relations that are established are equally pell-mell. That is why there is such a disharmony and imbalance in the normal individual. A seeker, as one who tries to regulate his life in accord with an ideal, has perforce to impose some kind of order on the functioning of his faculties, and on the way in which the mind coordinates the contacts to which he is exposed or which he chooses. And this is where concentration is indispensable.

Concentration, broadly speaking, means a willed use of a faculty with which we are concerned at a given moment. Speaking in the context of the yoga which we are considering, however, concentration has a more particular connotation. It means the gathering of our thought from its involvement in the many-sided flow of mental activities, and directing it toward a purpose, an objective that we have in view. It is a means by which thought is freed from its thraldom to the sense mind, to the restive logical mind which insists on pressing all experience into the mould of logic. The thoughts are gradually gathered, narrowed down into a thought, and in this thought so concentrated, one rises into the Real.

There are three powers or functions of concentration. First, by concentrating one's thought on an object or movement, one can force it to yield its contents, to be the object of one's knowledge. By sheer concentration upon an object, one makes an impact on the consciousness that is involved in the object and forces it to release the knowledge of its contents to the subject who concentrates upon it. Second, by concentrating the will, it is possible — if only one would persevere without succumbing to possible disappointments — to acquire what one does not have. If one marshalls one's will and directs it upon the object one wishes to acquire, one day the will asserts itself and the thing comes into the possession of the subject. There is another power of concentration. That is, by turning the concentration on a particular status of the being, it is possible to organise it and make it a real and permanent possession. Thus, for instance, if one is by nature a weakling and due to environmental influences is fearful and nervous, by concentrating upon a state of health and strength it is possible for a weakling to develop into a figure of strength, for a coward to grow into a hero.

There are three processes of concentration — concentration of thought, concentration of will, concentration of the being. The three may be utilised separately or together. This process of threefold concentration has certain well-marked gradations. There is first the step of purification; second, renunciation of activity that is foreign to the object of concentration; third, cessation of all activity which is not directly connected with the object of concentration. In concentration upon an object, first the consciousness mentally seizes it; thereafter, the problem is to hold it in one's attention; after holding it, the consciousness loses itself in the object, becomes one with the consciousness in the object.

This process, this discipline of concentration has been standardised and notably systematised in the raja yoga of Patanjali. As all of you are aware, the first two steps of this eightfold path of yoga are ones of purification; purification external and internal, cleanliness outer and inner. This process includes training the will Godward, disciplining the mind in the ways of holiness and purity. These two steps or limbs are indispensable indeed, whatever the yoga that one chooses. I have heard it lightly said that in our Integral Yoga, there is no need to absorb the preliminary limbs of raja yoga. The truth is to the contrary. Sri Aurobindo and the Mother take it for granted that one who chooses such a difficult ideal as the transformation of nature, the divinisation of oneself, has perforce gone through that preliminary discipline. It is assumed that one does not need to be put through that regimen. After all, the purification of the first two limbs, *yama* and *niyama*, is largely psychological, and unless one is psychologically equipped in that sense, it is impossible to make any headway in any yoga, much less the Integral Yoga which demands more of man than any other.

After one has purified oneself, eliminated the dross of inertia, *tamas*, proclivities toward lower movements, there comes the third step, posture, *asana*. There are as many as eighty possible postures, but they are not relevant to our purpose. Patanjali himself says that that posture is ideal in which one is at ease. The position in which one can hold oneself for a considerable length of time without pain or discomfort, the position which permits an uninterrupted flow of the life-force, the nerve-force into the nerve channels, is the ideal asana. Normally, all that is required is that one sits erect, without resting the head backwards or forwards. Therefore, during meditation or concentration, one shall not rest the head on a wall or chair. One may do it when one is contemplating or is in a relaxed condition, partly meditating, partly thinking. But serious concentration or meditation does not permit it. What is required is that the tip of the nose, the chest, and the spine are all in a straight line. In a number of Upanishads you will find this posture described as the ideal. These three points have to be in a line so that the breath goes from the head to the abdomen in a straight and direct manner; there is then no dissipation of life-energy.

Posture achieved, next there is the regulation of breath. There is an intimate connection between breathing and mental activity. When the mind is restless or furiously active, the breathing also is fast. Similarly, when the breathing is quick or hard, the mind is agitated. So the ancients discovered that by regulating the breath, one can regulate the flow of activities in the mind. They asked the seeker to gradually slow down the rate of breathing. As one slows it and establishes a rhythm in the incoming and outgoing breath, the workings of the mind, the flow of thoughts, fall into a certain pattern. The mind comes under control. This principle of regulation of thought by regulation of breath was developed into a fine science called *pranayama*, the elongation of breath. That science in its entirety has more than yogic results, and is a different topic into which we need not enter now.

The posture taken, the mind brought into minimum control by the regulation of breathing, the next step is to withdraw the mental faculties — the process called *pratyahara* in the ancient science — which are normally spread out in a hundred directions, and turn them inwards: not to allow them to gather food outside, to orient the mental faculties toward oneself and give them food within. This turning inward of the sense mind, of the cognising mind, is the next step. Once all the outspread mental faculties are gradually gathered and turned inward, they are massed and directed upon the object of concentration. It may be a name, it may be a form, it may be a sound. All the mental energies and faculties are gathered around that object, and are narrowed and narrowed, made to converge on that idea or form or sound. That is concentration.

In the very nature of things, it is not possible to maintain the tension of this state of concentration for long. With their fine knowledge of human psychology and capacities, the ancients prescribed that once the whole consciousness is brought together at a point, held for a while on the object of concentration, the next step is to release that gathered consciousness on the theme of the object. The mind is to be allowed to flow — in thoughts or ideas concerned with and governed by that object. Concentration gradually flows into meditation. From fixation, there is a gradual, controlled, well-directed movement in terms of the chosen theme. So, the mind is first freed from outer objects and brought to bear on an inner object; thereafter, thought is allowed to flow. As thought flows on the subject, gradually the mind acquires the character of the object meditated upon. It becomes one with it. And when all external existence is put aside and all internal consciousness is merged in the object, that marks the first stage of what is called samadhi, trance.

There is first the awareness that one is the knower and the object is the known. Gradually the consciousness of the distinction between the knower and known fades till the knower no longer is, only the object is; one loses oneself in the object. If, for instance, one chooses the theme of the Divine as love, when one brings the mind into focus and thinks of divine love, one ultimately comes to the essence of God as love. What love is, and how God manifests the qualities of love are parts of the process of analysing and understanding for oneself the implication of conceiving of the Divine as love. As one thinks of it, the process moves from the mind to the heart, from the heart to the rest of the being, so that not only is the mind full of the concept, but there is a spontaneous ebullition of love for God, of love for all, God in all. There is either a simultaneous or a successive experience of love in the mind and love in the heart. The very body exudes through its pores the vibrations of love. When you come into the presence of such a person, you feel warmed, you feel like loving everyone and all orders of creation. You see a tree or shell or person, and love flows from you. You don't need to force yourself to do it or imagine it. In the presence of divine love, you cannot but love whatever comes in the ambience of your consciousness.

Similarly, if one conceives of the Divine as power, one first understands the power aspect of the Divine, followed by an infusion of strength and power into one's being. These are successive steps or, as I said, simultaneous happenings in effective concentrations.

Concentration naturally needs — at any rate in the beginning — some support. One may choose a thought, a form, or a name. It is understood that whichever one selects, it is only the starting point, it is a springboard to soar or to delve into that which is behind the thought, the form, or the name. The name stands for something, the form symbolises some reality, thought is a projection of a greater reality than what is translated in the mental figure. So, in using them, the attempt is always to get beyond what one begins with.

It is understood that these practises are not superstitions. Dry philosophers may pride themselves and in the vanity of their knowledge say that repetition of a name, *japa*, or a mantra, is superstitious. Yet the validity of this practise is a fact of spiritual experience, capable of verification by anyone who takes the necessary steps therefor. Sri Aurobindo has written very highly of the symbolic word *OM* as a sure means of soaring out of the phenomenal into the Real. One of the classical Upanishads, the Mandukya, is devoted to a systematic exposition of the components of this sound — OM or AUM. It speaks of the sound as consisting of three parts: the first releasing vibrations that are relevant to the waking condition and the outer world; the second relating to the subtler world of dream, where things are planned, organised, and given subtle shape before being projected into the material; the third relating to where things are in a seed state, the sleeping condition. The waking condition, the dream state, the sleep state, and all together — AUM — rising in a potent sound into that which exceeds all the states, into the transcendent, the fourth stage.

So if one repeats this charged word, in the course of time the whole being quietens. The restless energies fall into a certain silence, and one begins to be liberated into infinity. OM is the one such word that does not need to be communicated by a guru. It is very good indeed if a guru imparts it, but even otherwise it is, it has become, a self-existent mantra. Millions have repeated it and added their force of consciousness to the sound vibrations of the word. And OM, you must remember, is the nearest approximation in human sound — sound which can be received by the physical ear on the earth plane — to the primordial sound or vibration, *nada*, which is said to have issued forth when the creative consciousness first stirred into movement before this manifestation emerged from the bosom of the eternal. So by repeating that word, one reforges a link with that primordial vibration where the existence is infinite, the consciousness is luminous, and the bliss is ever-flowing.

That is the importance of OM. There are indeed other words, particularly in the Tantras, called seed-letters or -sounds, which establish links with their relevant cosmic powers, or smaller deities or godlings; but we need not go into that subject now. And, when you concentrate on a thought, a form, a name or sound, the objective must always be to reach behind it, for they each sum up certain characteristics of the reality. Such a thought or name or sound is a power; such a form is a symbol; through them you can establish contact with the reality for which they stand. And in the process of concentration, these have a capital use.

By whichever means, one persists and traverses the whole gamut of samadhi experience. Samadhi means a gathered state of consciousness in which the consciousness is one with the object concentrated upon. There is no movement, even the seed-movement is not present. This is the highest state, where everything falls silent; one is just what one has concentrated upon. It is in that state — as though in the still, limpid water of a lake — that the reality reflects itself. That indeed is the goal of the traditional yogas.

For us, who believe not only in liberation but in fulfillment in the world, it is necessary to normalise that state of trance in waking life in order to canalise the results of liberation into the world for its perfection. How is that to be done? One starts, again, with a bifurcation of consciousness. There is a frontal part, always active, throwing itself into the movement; and there is behind a status of consciousness which derives from that state of concentration where one reflects the higher reality. One receives without interruption a continuous infusion from the higher plane. So this waking state of samadhi, what the Gita calls the *sahaja*, natural, samadhi, is our objective. Concentration is a means; meditation is a means; samadhi is a means. The object is to normalise that highest state of consciousness we can reach and make real to ourselves in peak periods of concentration. Periods for this purpose are very much necessary till one carries that poise all twenty-four hours — working, sleeping, sitting, or walking. It is a moving consciousness established in the poise of the eternal that should be our object. How we are going to do it, what is the way to set about it, is what we will be discussing in our future meetings.

Any questions?

If one wants to know about a particular aspect of some object, how do you direct the concentration without destroying that concentration?

First one has a certain mental conception, right or not fully right. The train of thought is then directed with a will on that theme, without allowing the mind to stray. The first steps are always speculation, discrimination, rejection; in that way there is an exercise of the mental faculty exploring the possibilities, eliminating what is not likely. In every way, the consciousness is kept centred. And when a certain tenseness or poise is developed, it attracts a response from the higher plane where there is an intuitive knowledge. When the whole mind is gathered and ready to receive the relevant knowledge, a ray from that intuitive level touches the mind. To properly understand and interpret that communication, purification is required. Otherwise the mind tends to read into it its own ideas. To put it simply, one has first to create a climate for the true knowledge to manifest. Prepare the background, create the necessary atmosphere, keep the whole being tuned to that — and it is understood that there is a certain call in the heart for that knowledge to manifest — and the response is bound to come.

Which method of contemplation did Sri Aurobindo use to silence his mind?

Sri Aurobindo did not use the method of concentration. First, he was just asked to sit quiet, and he did; he simply obeyed the teacher. He was told: when you are quiet, you will see thoughts coming from outside — throw them out. Sri Aurobindo said it was a new idea to him — that thoughts could be coming from outside — and he wanted to see it; and immediately he saw thoughts coming with concrete impact from outside. And, with a will, he just threw them aside.

This operation continued for three days — watching the thoughts and throwing them out — till the silence fully established itself. This does not and cannot happen to everybody. It was the presence and the dynamism of the person who was sent to Sri Aurobindo by God that was responsible; and of course, his own unquestioning obedience to the guru. He did not use the process of concentration; he was just quiet, and did that which he was told. What happened was that the inner, the subtler layers of the mind came forward and there was absolute peace — a state which never left him thereafter. The brain apparatus fell silent; afterwards, the brain, as such, never operated. He explained that he never thought when he wrote; he was always conscious — whether it was a letter, the *Arya* or *The Life Divine* — that it was always from above the higher mind that things were coming. The brain was a channel, but never something that formed the thoughts.

So he did not arrive at silence or peace by concentration, but that can't be the rule. There are cases, no doubt, where people have stumbled upon silence without having to concentrate. Such cases can be explained by saying that in their previous birth they had arrived at that point of evolution where the silence of the mind or the being was nearing realisation, yet somehow it was not then completed, and some small incident or provocation is enough to light up that possibility in the present birth. When one hears of someone achieving realisation in five minutes, this is why. A realisation which had failed to fructify in the previous incarnation is fulfilled in the present.

Sri Aurobindo was not an evolving being — as we are — who had to do yoga and achieve spiritual evolution or liberation. He had to find and forge a new way, for a new goal. And that is why, as a representative of earth, of humanity, he did what he did. Even as the Mother today is subjecting herself to the process of transformation not as an individual but as a representative of the earth-being, carrying all the obstructions and resistances that are still in earth-consciousness, earth-nature, and exposing them to the force that is acting, Sri Aurobindo's yoga was done more as a representative than as a seeker.

Is it better to concentrate on one thing continually, day after day, until it is realised, or is it all right to change?

One cannot be rigid in these matters, because certain things fall away after their use is over. I may be repeating a mantra or concentrating upon a particular form, but if that exercise has fulfilled its purpose and given me the necessary poise or experience, it tends to drop off by itself. One cannot stick to something which has outlived its purpose. This is a dynamic yoga, with fresh possibilities and horizons coming every day. It is not as if we have one limited objective of seeing what is behind a particular form; if that is the objective, one can't give it up till one has come to the "other side" of the form. But for us that is not the aim. We use these things as aids and supports for the gathering of our consciousness and for delivering it into the hands of the yoga-force that is to achieve the change in us. We certainly do not expect that individually we will work out the whole process of transformation in ourselves. We have our part to play till the surrender is complete, the receptivity is fully organised, the ego is eliminated, and the psychic is awakened. Thereafter neither the process of concentration nor meditation nor samadhi is necessary. There is a natural efflorescence of spiritual development because it is something else that takes charge. We have only to support and collaborate from our lower end.

Many yogas, in India particularly, make concentration and meditation ends in themselves, and that is where they fall short. Worship is not an end in itself, doing japa a thousand times is not an end in itself. All these things thereby become mechanical; and the moment a thing becomes mechanical, that is a signal that you have to stop it. Unless you can revivify a process by a fresh breath of aspiration, it is useless spiritually to persist with a practice that has ceased to be living.

One can think of Mother in her wholeness, or one can think of Mother in her aspects – her peace or power, for example. Is it better sometimes to think only of her peace rather than of her wholeness? How does one know what to limit one's concentration to?

To put it in another way, the approach to the Divine is twofold: it can be either in its personal or impersonal aspect. The impersonal approach is when you conceive of the Divine, or for us Mother, who is divine for us, and adore her as love, compassion, grace, peace, joy. One can think of her according to the situation, to the difficulty, to the need of the hour. But, when she is available in a personal form, and if we can establish a link — by love, surrender, devotion, adoration — with the person of the Mother, then all these impersonal aspects of hers respond according to our need without our having to concentrate upon that aspect. If I am disturbed or agitated, if only I think of Mother with love, remember and call her, that which is necessary to heal my agitation — the peace, the calm — comes unasked. Her face, her frontal person releases an immense reservoir of divine energies, an outflow of consciousness, in whatever aspect you pray for. Both are good, but to think of her in a personal way is quicker, more satisfying and spiritually rewarding.

What would you advise in a work situation, in Auroville, where the concentration has to be on the work itself, and yet one wants always to refer it to the Divine and make it an occasion for inner progress?

This idea of progressing towards the Divine, of growing in one's consciousness through work need not be overly dwelt upon during the course of work. Before starting, one offers, dedicates, prays, aspires. Thereafter, the bulk of the concentration must be on the work. The character of the work is different once you dedicate it. You have to concentrate upon making the work itself more and more perfect. The inner being, which has dedicated itself at the outset, draws the necessary guidance, light, and energies and pours them into you as you are working. So much so that the guidance is automatic, spontaneous. There is no tiredness, normally, up to a certain point. One part is always linked. That is why there has to be a bifurcation of consciousness at every level. When you do work, you have to be concentrated only on work; but the whole basis is different in consecrated work. And you should have the trust that you will be guided. When a challenge presents itself, then is the time to pause a little and look for guidance. There in order to catch the right guidance, purification is presupposed — that you don't allow your own preferences and egoistic considerations to interfere or to parade under the guise of divine guidance. As Sri Aurobindo has said, the vital is a great charlatan, and he can very well put on the cloak of the Divine.

It is a question of sincerity. A sincere work, even — up to a certain stage — wrongly done, can be spiritually rewarding. But there must be sincerity. Somewhere, at some stage, the guidance comes through someone or through your own awakening, and you correct yourself.

4

Renunciation

We have discussed the role of purification in the yoga of knowledge. Purification not only of the emotions and impulsions of the heart and the vital, but also of the different layers and faculties of the mind, in order that the system may be opened to the working of higher faculties like intuition, illumination, and others. We next spoke of the indispensability of concentration and observed that mere purification without concentration could lead to a sterile passivity. If we believe in the yoga of action and change, it is indispensable that concentration be brought to bear on the area that has been subjected to purification. We also observed that purification and concentration are not so much successive processes as simultaneous ones. As purification proceeds, concentration becomes easier, unclogged by the impurities in the nerve channels; and as concentration develops, purification becomes easier, because we know exactly where the pressure is to be applied and all the energies are massed together to achieve the purpose in view.

These two processes together — purification and concentration — are likened by Sri Aurobindo to the right hand, and the role of renunciation to the left hand of the yoga of knowledge. He calls renunciation the left hand not, indeed, to reduce its value, but to emphasise that its role is largely negative. Concentration and purification build up in ourselves the truth of existence, consciousness, bliss, illumination — of all that we associate with the Divine. They build, they organise, they confirm the higher value. But renunciation is concerned with removing the obstructions, plucking out the roots of ignorance and falsehood that lie deep in our nature.

Renunciation deals with the disassociation of ourselves from all that stands in the way of progress. It is a negative but an indispensable process that every seeker has to undergo on some plane or another.

Renunciation has acquired quite a different significance in certain traditions, particularly in Asia. Renunciation is associated with the rejection of life — life as it is lived in the world. It is pointed out that there is something radically wrong with the life of the world, and it is best to excise that area from oneself should one desire spiritual liberation. There is nothing in common between the devious life in the world and the royal path of the spiritual life. We are told that, "Straighten however you will the tail of the dog, it is bound to return to its crooked position." All steps of ethics, morality, religion have not succeeded in transforming life. Life is only a stumbling block in the way of aspiration. And, logically, we reject what stands in our way; we withdraw — either physically into a cave or forest or into ourselves — keeping out of our ambit the life of the world, and there we work out our salvation.

This is one reason why renunciation of the world is called for. Buddhism and Hinduism are replete with splendid instances of renunciation from gallant spirits who have walked out in the midst of the splendour of life, hearkening to the call of the spirit. Another reason why renunciation of the world has been popular is the almost exclusive preoccupation with personal salvation, release from the rounds of life and death, and an exit into a blissful beyond or into an indefinable and indescribable nonexistence.

Thirdly, there is a joy in renunciation for its own sake, there is as much joy in asceticism as in enjoyment; it gives as much of a thrill, as much strength, pleasure, and excitement. There is a feeling of having done something and of having arrived when one practices asceticism. That is why in Indian mythology you hear of titans and demon-kings practicing austerities and symbolically doing penance for hundreds of years, renouncing enjoyment and pleasure, renouncing the senses, because they enjoy asceticism. From the spiritual standpoint, both uninhibited enjoyment and uncontrolled asceticism occupy the same place on the scale of values.

The fourth reason is failure in life; weakness in nature and weakness of spirit to face the problem of life and solve it, to square it with the needs of the soul. The inability of the weak human spirit to meet this challenge is also responsible for the popular acceptance of renunciation as a way of spiritual life.

It is clear that for the seeker of the integral path, this type of renunciation is out of the question. For him, life indeed acts as a challenge. If life is contaminated, he is called upon to purify it, to restore to it its original purity and to uplift it. He cannot look upon life as an evil dream, as a delirium of the soul; he is called upon to realise life in the world as a manifestation of the Divine. Personal salvation, as such, has no appeal to the seeker of the integral path. Personal liberation is a necessary and an indispensable step towards perfection — liberation, not so much from the rounds of life and death, but from the hold of ignorance, falsehood, and the lower nature in order to enter into the belt of the supernature.

He does not value salvation in order to enjoy the divine bliss for himself; he has a heart that beats in tune with the hearts of the millions who are suffering still. His ears still listen to the cry coming from below. He considers it beneath his dignity and stature to work for his own salvation, leaving the rest of the world, his brethren, as they are. Weakness of spirit, the inability to face the challenge of life is foreign to him — or at any rate, it ought to be foreign — because he does not depend upon his own strength.

The very first step that he takes as he launches upon the quest for perfection is to lay himself open to the action of a mighty force of the Divine. He makes himself an instrument, a working ground for the operations of a force higher than his own. There is nothing too difficult, nothing insurmountable to the force and the power to which he opens himself. For all these reasons, he does not accept the gospel of renunciation of the world.

It has been a tragedy in India that during the decadent curve of her civilization, when the force of life ebbed, renunciation as a part of or as a step to higher life came to be accepted. That is why there are institutions promoting renunciation, preparing people for renunciation. It is because of that that India has lagged behind in the battle for the fruits of life. The time has come indeed when India has been slowly awakening; with the arrival on the scene of Vivekananda, the soul of India stirred. It has realised that mere renunciation is cowardice. Vivekananda called upon his countrymen to renounce weakness and poverty of the spirit, and to take with both hands the riches of the earth and the riches of the spirit.

Sri Aurobindo continues this tradition, enlarges upon it and adds a new dimension; and he points out that what is to be renounced is within ourselves. We do not have to renounce anything outside; as a matter of fact it is not ours to renounce. What obtains on earth — natural riches, material prosperity, affluence — all belongs to the Lord. "All is for habitation by the Lord" — this is the injunction of the first verse of one of the oldest Upanishads of India. You have no right to it; you have no right to renounce it, much less to claim it. The true renunciation is inner.

What is to be renounced in each individual? First, attachment and desire — attachment of the senses to their objects, desire of the vital and the physical-vital for enjoyment. To cling to things of the world, to appropriate things for oneself, are movements to be renounced. The drive of the senses to appropriate things, to hold things in their grasp and to brood over them when they are not accessible — that is, to live in and dwell upon them — forms the attachment. This attachment and the wish to appropriate larger and larger segments of life, to exercise proprietorship over them, is desire. This attachment and desire of the senses bind one to the earth. That is why one is called upon to renounce this attachment, to renounce desire.

Second, the habit of assertion of will in thought and action must be overpassed. Each one has his pet ideas as to what should be done, how things should be thought out, what ideas are right, and he insists that these must form the mould in which all thinking should flow; all must adopt his system. This attachment to and assertion of one's own preference and one's own orientation to thinking, and after thinking, to action in the world, claiming superiority, monopoly of truth, exclusiveness to one's own approach or designed mould — these should be renounced.

Third, there is the central egoism. The ego is the linchpin which holds together the whole of the lower, human life, attached to the world. Everything, from the smallest to the largest consideration — from food to meditation — is governed, directed, conducted with reference to the ego, to how it affects oneself. With anything that happens, at home or elsewhere, the first reaction is, "How does it affect me?" If today the dollar is devalued by ten percent, the first reaction is, "By how much do my dollar holdings come down?"; if there is a storm and rain, "How is my house going to be affected?" We rarely think of what is going to happen to the community, to the whole collectivity. This sense of I-ness and my-ness is the bane; it is to be eradicated. Egoism is the powerful center of the whole nonspiritual, unspiritual life.

These are the three things — attachment and desire, assertion of will in thought and action, and the central egoism that dominates the whole pattern of life — that are to be renounced.

In this process, the seeker of the integral path knows that

when he rejects attachment and desire, there is no self-denial. There is only denial of ignorance. He knows, as Sri Aurobindo graphically describes, that attachment is only egoism in love. In the lower hemisphere, one claims a certain exclusive proprietorship on the object of love; one will be hurt if the loved one were to equally love another. Spiritual love would permit, certainly, loving of all; it is a sign of lower love when there is a claim — explicit or implicit — of exclusive possession of the one loved. This is the badge of human love. In spiritual love, on the contrary, the whole direction is towards expansion; love prospers, love grows, love delights in the measure in which it spreads. Actually, limitation, restriction, hurts the soul that loves.

Most of you were not in the ashram twenty or twenty-five years ago. The Mother used to meet all the disciples, devotees, and visitors, and one could observe the different reactions from people. Those who really received her love as divine love and loved her from the heart with a certain purity of self-giving, enjoyed seeing her loving others, pouring her compassion and love on everyone who came to her. They felt uplifted, elevated. To sit there and watch her receive people was itself a sadhana, was itself a yogic lesson. One's whole being would expand; people used to feel widened. One wouldn't know one's limits — whether there was a top to the head, or where the body ended. There was a feeling of expansion.

But there were those who in their consciousness had limited the Mother's love to themselves. They would feel jealous when they saw Mother smiling a little more, spontaneously, to others. They would get angry and write letters to Sri Aurobindo saying that the Mother loved someone else more than them. Sri Aurobindo wrote countless letters disabusing the minds of sadhaks of this illusion. But ultimately it told on the Mother's body; and when the *pranams* had to be stopped, Sri Aurobindo wrote to the effect that she had brought down the divine love and tried to share it, to give it to all, but the inmates started pulling her down to their human level, and that strain was too much on her, she had to withdraw.

All this I mention just to point out the difference between the attachment in human love and the freedom, the elevation of divine love. When the seeker rejects attachment and desire, it is not that he rejects compassion or that he rejects divine love, it is not that he becomes indifferent or aloof to the cry of humanity. He embraces it from a higher level, and perhaps a more effective level. He does not need to declare that he will not accept salvation till the last man on earth is saved. The very problem he sets before himself — that of transformation — is such that nothing is complete unless all is complete. Until the last knot of egoism and falsehood in cosmic nature is loosened and untied — not cut, that's not the Mother's way — the reign of falsehood and egoism in oneself and in others cannot be said to have been finally ended.

I was reading yesterday a message given by the Mother that the only remedy for falsehood in the world is for each individual to cure whatever in his consciousness contradicts the divine presence. It is by meeting squarely the challenge of falsehood in oneself that one can solve the problem of the cosmic falsehood. That is because, like truth, falsehood — which is a deliberate deformation and perversion of truth — is also spread wide in the universe. It is one body and a dent made at one point affects the whole structure. It is not possible for us to attack and dissolve falsehood outside ourselves as easily as it is to isolate, study, and eliminate it within ourselves. That is why the Mother always stresses change, the resolution of knots, in oneself first. That gives us a hold to deal with the cosmic problem more easily. It is impossible to eliminate darkness and obscurity elsewhere unless one eliminates it in oneself.

This rejection of all that is undivine, the disassociation of ourselves from all that holds us down, is real renunciation. Giving up these things from ourselves in order that the finding of the Self may be truer and greater.

As promised, I will now give in more detail the background of the Mother's reply to a letter written by a friend here regarding "hippies".

The letter, indeed, summed up all that thinking people have felt on the subject, and it was remarkable for the frankness with which the sentiments were expressed. I took the letter to the Mother, and by the time I finished reading just the first paragraph, she opened her eyes and started telling me her answer.

She said that, for our purpose, those who are unclean and take drugs are to be kept out — it does not matter by what name you call such people. But if they are clean, if they don't take drugs, even if they wear unconventional clothes and have long hair, she said, "I welcome them with open arms."

I was struck by this because at the end of the letter the writer had written, "Are they not your children? Won't you welcome them with open arms?" I had not read that portion, but still she repeated it.

Someone present immediately asked, "But Mother, you are saying unconventional clothes are permissible, then people . . ." She said, "I do not care for your conventions. I am out to break conventions."

And then she went on to explain why she objects to uncleanliness and drugs. She said that in India, particularly, unless one is clean, one is susceptible to all kind of diseases, especially leprosy. Second, she said that drugs lower the consciousness whereas our object is to raise the consciousness. Drugs induce vital experiences that many mistake to be spiritual experiences, and they go astray. Then she added that even if a person is habitually unclean, even if a person has been taking drugs, if he says that he will be clean here, will stop taking drugs, then a chance must be given. This is a place where people must come to change, and those who want to change will be given a chance.

Immediately after speaking to Mother, I wrote down what she had said, because I knew the implications. I then went back and read out to her what I had recorded; she listened very carefully and said it was accurate. Though it was in answer to a personal letter, I mentioned that it could be circulated amongst all who are concerned about this matter, and I hope it has answered any doubts.

Two or three days thereafter, I was given for reply a series of questions on the subject of hippies by the journal *Sri Aurobindo's Action.* I have kept a copy of my answers which I thought I should share with you in order that you may know my mind and, if I am not correctly informed, in order that I could be corrected in these matters, as in all matters.

The first question was: *"What is meant by the word 'hippie'?"*

My reply: "A hippie is, in current usage, one who is in revolt against society, against its established customs, norms, standards. This revolt expresses itself outwardly in his discarding the forms of living that are normally accepted. Inwardly, he ceases to believe in established religion and questions the very basis of authority in every field of life."

"Has the growth of hippies some relation with the youth unrest?"

"As a matter of fact, the unrest is not confined to the young. There is a universal unrest, inevitable at a stage of evolutionary transition such as at present, when old values are breaking down under the pressure of the forward movement of the evolutionary consciousness on earth, and new ones have not yet formed roots. Youth unrest is really a part of this ferment, though the spirit of change is naturally more articulate in the young than in the old."

"Can the hippies have a place in the new society that is emerging?"

"In the measure in which this movement sheds its negative elements, eliminates the abuses that have crept in, and increases its positive elements, it can certainly be a factor for progress in the new direction. Denial and rejection of old values is to give place to the cultivation, promotion and establishment of a new truth that can add a fresh dimension to the being of man. Necessarily, dissipation, drug abuse and the like, which bring down the consciousness, weaken the will, close the doors to the advent of a diviner consciousness and drag man into the glittering wilderness of the vital, before landing him in ruins — physical, mental, moral, and spiritual — must be rejected without compromise, before the positive contribution can start."

This is my considered reading of the situation.

The word hippie itself has acquired so many connotations. Actually, we are all hippies — some on the physical plane, some, like me, on the mental plane. Till I arrived at a certain mental conviction that, "This is the truth for me, this is the way", I was indeed a mental hippie. I would consider so many ideas, think of them today, give them up tomorrow and take another, continually changing and experimenting without sticking to anything; are we not all, at some stage or another, mental hippies? This hippie phenomenon has drawn attention only when it has come down to and expressed itself on the physical plane. It is an eternal phenomenon of trying and changing, not sticking to a thing, giving up old things, trying new things. As everything else, this too has been projected onto the physical plane for correction, for adaptation, and for restoration in the true values.

Any questions?

I feel the vibration in the ashram is getting so suspicious against any young person not dressed all in white and looking very saintly, and I'm very sad that the prejudice against any nonconvention is promoted in Mother's name, while Mother says, "I am out to break conventions."

In Mother's name, so many things are going on in the ashram, in Auroville, and elsewhere also. When I ask Mother about these things, she just shrugs her shoulders. She refuses to take action. She believes in inner action and inner pressure for change.

Everybody really knows the truth of the matter. Those who think and whose opinions matter, the healthy sections of ashram society, know very well what Mother wants. And be assured that as long as there are elements loyal to Mother, loyal to Truth, no injustice will be done. We are here to seek for the Truth and the Spirit, and whatever the human maneuverings, things will right themselves. Life has to be a series of balancings, temporary compromises, acceptance of lesser evils to avoid greater ones.

There is a similar prejudice against itinerant sannyasins who come to the ashram. They say, "What kind of ashram is this? All over India, wherever we go to an ashram, we are taken care of, and here in this ashram we are denied accomodations." I remember one particular sannyasi who came with one or two disciples and asked if they could stay. Mother has given me the discretion to accept such people as guests for a few days. I told them they could stay for a day as our guests. But when he started complaining, lecturing and posturing, I politely excused myself and withdrew the offer. Then he turned to his disciples and said in Hindi, thinking that I wouldn't understand, "These are worldly people."

The institution of *sannyas* has been abused and degraded. Similarly, the genuine hippie movement has been subjected to certain abuses and degradations in India, and that is why opinion has been roused against it. Bad elements masquerading as hippies have given a bad name. Otherwise, India is known for its hospitality and would never think of shutting out any person simply because he is a hippie. In line with our tradition, our doors are open; and much more so in the ashram.

In a collective society, some rules, I suppose, are inevitable. Individual discretion and tact can avert many unpleasant situations.

I tell you sincerely that the unhappiest person in the ashram over the whole situation is Mother herself. I know this to be true. Her way is different; she doesn't believe in outer, enforced discipline, in rules and regulations, in permit cards and such things. But we have forced her to come down, in certain ways, to the administrative level of functioning as in present human society, and we have made necessary all these rules. Otherwise, for instance, she said that the four things mentioned in the charter are enough for Auroville, no rules or regulations should be necessary. But what has happened, how many regulations have had to be made since then? Why should they be needed? If all of us really believe in the growth of consciousness, in adjustment of consciousness, in functioning on the level of consciousness, why do we want rules? Why can't we make adjustments between ourselves? The problem is the rigidity of the mind and attachment to ideas; each one thinks that his understanding is right and everyone else must follow him.

At times Mother is really alarmed. Why are all these things of the old type of society, like rules and regulations, present in Auroville? She doesn't want them to be here. She could not prevent them in some ways in the ashram; and she had been hoping to realise her dream here in Auroville. My soul weeps when I see her unhappy, so indrawn, and conceding things with a sad gesture. If at ninety-four she still has to fight against the human obstinacy to stick to its ignorance, what hope is there for humanity?

She told me once that ever since she was five she has been conscious of the work for which she came. Ever since then she has seen a light that guides her. She doesn't make a single decision unless she receives a sign. She has no personal objective in life. She has no need to retain her present body and suffer all its old age infirmities; none at all. It is for humanity that she undergoes all that torturous pain. When are we going to respond to her call, to her demands? Well, each individual can start in himself.

I was asked the other day, "How can we build up Mother's consciousness in ourselves?" The reply is straightforward: each time you meet someone, first think of Mother, and then act; at each impulse or each impact, in each circumstance, first think of her, and then respond. In that way a center of reference to the Mother's consciousness is built up, and her consciousness takes a permanent position in your being so that there is thereafter an automatic action. To organise and establish her consciousness, you must start by referring every little thing to her; don't do a thing without thinking of her. One need not necessarily pray for guidance, just to remember her is enough. This immediately forges the link and draws the needed guidance, because there is already in each one of us an emanation of hers. She has said that the moment she sees a person and there is an interchange, an emanation reaches out from her and lives with the person thereafter.

To illustrate: I met recently a remarkable visitor in one of our guest houses. A middle-aged man, he does not know a word of English and I don't know much of his language. Anyway, he asked me if he could see Mother, and I arranged it; then he gave a long letter for her. In it he explained that after coming here, without his realising it, he started doing yoga. He said he has begun to feel calm and peaceful in his mind, but his heart does not open. He feels something like an opening only when he sits before the photos of Sri Aurobindo and the Mother, but it doesn't last long. So he asked Mother if she could help. Secondly, he said that he is full of enthusiasm for the ideal of transformation and for what is going on here, and would like to communicate this message of hope to all his friends in Paris when he returns. But at the same time, he has a fear that when he goes and mixes with his old friends, he might lose what he has gained here. So he is in a dilemma and asked Mother what he is to do.

When I told this to Mother, she said, "Tell him the Force won't go; he must not lose faith."

Normally, I repeat to her what I hear so that I am sure I have heard it correctly, so I told her, "Yes, Mother, I shall tell him 'The Force won't go; he must not lose faith.'"

She said, "No, no, that's not it. The Force won't go *even if* he loses faith."

She added that what happens when people lose faith is that the Force continues, only they do not feel it. There is a veil drawn. The Force won't go in any event; you may not feel it if you lose faith, but the Force won't go.

Her emanation which dwells in each of us, doesn't leave us. It is man who withdraws from Grace, not the Grace that withdraws from man.

5

The Synthesis of the Disciplines of Knowledge

We have now discussed at some length the role of concentration and renunciation in spiritual life. Whichever path one chooses, — the path of works, devotion or knowledge — renunciation and concentration are to be applied in the way that corresponds to the distinctive line of development of those yogas.

Thus, for instance, in the path of works what is to be renounced is the ego-sense, the sense of the doer, the way of doing works that would forge chains of karma. The concentration has to be on the spirit of consecration, the spirit of surrender, and the process of working it out in detail. In the path of love what is to be renounced is what passes for love, the life and demands of the unpurified senses, whether in the realm of the material world or of the spirit. There must be concentration on a sustained and increasing purification of the being, cultivation of devotion leading to adoration, adoration melting into love. In the path of knowledge, renunciation lies in the rejection of what is not true, of what is not the self. Concentration is on the forging of union, of identity with the Self. How precisely these twin principles — positive and negative, passive and active — are to be harnessed in the path of knowledge is the theme of our present discussion.

The aim of the traditional path of knowledge is the discovery of the Self. At present, living in ignorance, the relations of the life of man with his true self are based on a certain falsity. Man is not aware of his true self, nor is he aware of the true self of others. His actions and movements — physical, vital, mental and emotional — are based on certain *ad hoc* arrangements arrived at between executive Nature and the surface soul. It is the aim of the path of knowledge to break through this system of false relations basing our everyday life and to arrive at the right relation between ourselves and our Self, between ourselves and the Self of all. As things stand at present, we are inclined to feel that we are the physical body. Intellectually we may know that we are not the body, that we are something else possessing the body. But in practice the identification with the body is so complete that man is just a physical creature subject to the changes of moods, needs and other movements of the material body. This relation has to be set right.

Similarly, there is the individuation of life-force in each person. One identifies oneself with the particular formation of life-force in his own body. He forgets that what he calls his own life-force is but a current, a wave in the ocean of the life-energy that is flowing in the universe. So too, one thinks that his mind is all. He forgets that his mind is but one part of a large and infinite Mind that is looming over this living, material creation.

This identification of the being of man, as far as he is conscious, with the physical body, with the life-force activating the physical body and with the mind pretending to lead this body and life-force completely falsifies the whole life-relation. It is the first lesson of the path of knowledge that one is not the body, one is not the life-force, one is not the mind. The process is twofold, negative and positive. Negatively, one affirms to oneself, "I am not this, I am not that". As one continually affirms one's freedom from the constrictions of the body, mind and life, grooves are formed in one's consciousness that attract the movement that will liberate one from lower nature. One becomes free from involvement in the body and in the triple bondage, first on levels of which one is not conscious, thereafter on levels of which one is half-conscious, and ultimately on levels of which one is conscious. It is a long process which has to be worked out in detail. At each step this dissociation from the body, the life-force and the mind has to be put into operation. The mind must be freed from its total identification with the body and its needs. The mind has got into the habit for instance of suffering with the body that suffers, feeling joy with the body that enjoys — in short, the mind in most has no independent existence from the life in the body. It is connected as a wheel to the chariot. It imagines it is leading but it is not. In the present economy of nature organised on the basis of ignorance and ego, the mind is a slave. The soul is not yet awake.

It is the business of the path of knowledge to teach the mind to separate itself from its involvement and identification with what it is not; this is done by the negative process of rejection, of renunciation, to educate it in a more positive way, to turn it to its own truth. As the mental being or *purusha* — the being that presides over the mental realm — is freed from the hectic movements of lower nature, it tends to fall quiet; then the process must be initiated of teaching the mind that "I *am* the self". The self that is aloof, the self that is the witness and the self that is the master — these are its three gradations. The mind should be trained, educated, orientated towards the self, of which it is a projection on the mental level.

As a result of this progressive affirmation of its inner identity with the self, the mind puts on another character, the character of the liberated self. As man the mental being dissociates himself from the material frame and identifies himself more and more with the witness self, with the silent self, there is an inevitable tendency to withdraw from action, to retreat, to renounce life: to stop the false account but not yet to open the right account. Sri Aurobindo says that this liberation from the necessity of having to work in the round of Nature is indispensable. The power to desist from action is also necessary, but certainly it is not at all advisable or called for to retire from action. For after all, action is the characteristic of the manifestation of the divine reality.

The seeker has to act, but act in an uninvolved way. It will not do to make himself a prisoner of a fad of inaction. One must not be bound to action, but also one shall not be bound to inaction. A stage arrives when, from this poise in the witness self, in the silent observing self, action and inaction cease to be different. It is something else that acts, carries out the sanction, the will — a will that does not emanate from one's personal self, but is reflected in the Self from on high. This state has to be cultivated and normalised.

For the seeker of the traditional path of knowledge, it is enough to reject the world as a circumstance of a false relation between Nature and its Lord. He escapes, or he seeks to escape into the beyond, whether the beyond is full of bliss or an ineffable nothingness, *nirvana*. There he reaches his end; the traditional path of knowledge leads to this liberation. But for a seeker of the integral goal, this is not the way. The world continues to exist, people continue to suffer, ignorance and death continue to rule, whatever the number of those who scale the heights of the Spirit and pass into the beyond.

It is the characteristic of the Integral Yoga that one has to utilise the gains of the path of knowledge, of the state of liberation that one achieves, for effecting the liberation of the collective nature from its thraldom to ignorance and falsehood. One has to bring this consciousness to bear upon the situation. He realises the self within; he learns as a result of the pressure of the knowledge that is real to him that the same self is also the Self of all. He realises that the Self within him, at a certain level, is the lord of not only his own nature but all Nature. And the Lord of all is also the absolute reality, the *Brahman* that transcends all thought.

In fact, it is the transcendent that projects itself, collectively, as the universal Self and individually as the individual self. The one who is liberated in the path of knowledge is not only free from involvement in nature, but he attains a perfect identity — step by step — with this triple self-formulation of the Absolute in the world.

There are, indeed, a number of things in the traditional way of knowledge that a seeker of this path can draw upon. Nobody leaps into the beyond with one step. In Vedanta different gradations of the self are recognised. First they speak of the universal Self, the Self that has become all these existences. This is the Self of the waking condition; the Self of which we in our waking state are parts. Next they speak of the subtler, the perceptively creative soul, the Divine Self that creates on a subtler level forms which later take material shape on earth. He is called the dream Self. All of us, when we dream, pass into a state where we are parts of the universal dream-Self. Still more subtle there is what is called the sleep Self, the wise one, the *Prajna.* Above all the three there is the fourth Self, the absolute, transcendent.

These four selves are not separate selves ruling four different empires. Each one of us has these four levels, four planes of consciousness and being, and it is possible by developing the consciousness to realise our identity with them, to realise ourselves, to awaken ourselves on these four planes of existence — simultaneously at a certain level, successively at the frontal level. It is a comprehensive realisation to be awake on all four levels, to integrate the four levels of existence in one awakened, luminous consciousness.

The bits of knowledge, the processes that have been perfected in *jnanayoga*, the traditional path of knowledge, are useful provided we know how to utilise them. Renunciation, yes; rejection of the world, yes — but at a certain stage. Sri Aurobindo says that in the life of many a stage does come when things have to be absolutely renounced. Attachment to things is so strong in certain natures that a surgical operation becomes necessary. If you cannot untie the knot, as the

Upanishad puts it, you have to cut the knot. Untying the knot is the Mother's way. She never advises or undertakes a radical cutting off. With all her motherly patience, she unties the tangled knots, one by one; always with a smile, always with a consoling touch if the process hurts the person concerned.

In the Upanishad they speak of the knot of the heart, the *hridayagranthi*, where attachment and certain emotions keep the soul tied, behind a veil. It is easy enough to dissolve external knots, but the knots within have to be untied. Sri Aurobindo says that for some this untying is not possible. Because, either as a result of the past or of reckless living or of involvement in the present life, they are so much attached that some radical cutting off, *for some time*, is advisable.

It is understood that once the separation from the *prakriti*, from the lower nature, is effected, thereafter the soul, the true being, assumes its rightful control over nature. But before assuming control, one has to separate oneself from that which one would control. First separation, then assumption of control.

A wise rule is that of the Gita: austerities, if they be necessary, shall not be excessive. The Lord complains in the Gita that those who practise strenuous austerities, who deny food and drink to the body etc., deny experience to the soul in the world — they deny Him who is seated in the chamber of the heart. He says this titanic austerity, this *asuric tapasya* as it is termed in Sanskrit, offends the Lord who is seated in the temple of the heart. There are gentler ways, more becoming ways of leaving the animality of nature and growing into full manhood. The process has to be patient. One has, gently, to disengage oneself from the knots of the body, as also from the knots of the life-force.

Sri Aurobindo also makes a distinction between the life-force that supports the body, physical prana, and that part of the life-force which goes to support the mind, the psychic prana. First one has to withdraw from entanglement in the physical prana. When one releases oneself from attachment to the physical body, when one no more feels tied up with the little life-current that flows in one particular body, death loses its terror.

Sri Aurobindo calls death the badge of animality. And one who would rise above animalhood, arrive at full manhood and proceed towards his Godhead, has to wipe out this badge of animality.

Any questions?

You were talking about the four states. I had the impression that they exist in us simultaneously, all the time. Is it true that some part of us is always dreaming and some part always sleeping?

That is what I said. On a certain plane all four are simultaneously active and we can become conscious of them in an integrated way. But it is not on the surface. It is in the depths and on the heights behind the surface that they are all alive.

Is it this that we experience at night when we are asleep? Is that the type of sleep that is happening?

Yes. When we sleep, mostly we are in the realm of the dream Self.

There are certain Upanishads — perhaps you might read my *Essence of the Upanishads* — which describe how many senses are active in each state of consciousness. You see, for instance, there may be in the waking condition eighteen; in the dream condition fourteen, etc. They make a distinction and mention which senses are dormant, which senses are active in the different states.

When we sleep we don't go into that condition which is called the 'sleep'. It is only in certain trances, when the senses are absolutely dormant, that we pass into the consciousness that relates to the sleep Self. Normally when we sleep we are still on the dream level, only we are not conscious at the recording level. We say "I had a dreamless sleep". But to have a dreamless sleep, as the Mother once said, is a great feat. One arrives at it only in trance; when the whole consciousness is indrawn, organised, it falls naturally around the silent Self. But that comes only by yoga.

Then if we are conscious of these things, is it one of the possibilities to remain conscious through the experience of death?

If one is awake, if one's consciousness is organised, death does not make a difference. One passes through the experience of death as one passes through the gates of a house. Provided that during one's lifetime one has accustomed his multifold consciousness to the experience of moving from state to state or plane to plane of consciousness. He feels lighter, more powerful, larger. And that is why in spiritual history, in the lives of yogis, you find that they are more effective in their action on the world when they shed the physical instrument.

Why has Mother been relatively silent on Auroville recently?

Nowadays Mother doesn't express things as freely as she used to. She once explained that when things are expressed it immediately raises up so many hostile elements who say, "Oh, yes? I see, well let me show you." She said this was happening. That is why till a thing is realised, established beyond the possibility of reversal she does not wish to speak, and she asks all of us not to speak of anything in the process of growth. Not even to think aloud of it because this too raises certain vibrations. So she has not been expressing things freely.

All the while even when we are telling her things, reporting, her consciousness seems to be turned elsewhere.

I don't think the progress of Auroville is to be measured in terms of this many buildings coming up, this many people living here. She said if we are wanted to we could fill up the whole of Auroville with useless people in one night. She said it last month. But she said we have to be extremely careful, otherwise it will become an ordinary town. We do not want that to happen, so we have to be extremely careful in our choice of men, of things, of everything.

As far as I have understood, as far as I have known her reactions, she regards only the consciousness of people — how they react, how they act — rather than how much work is done in terms of bricks and mortar, of so many acres acquired, developed. But she can feel the breath of consciousness that is in each colony here, in each individual. And it is the duty of everyone, whether in the ashram or here, to see that for all that she has done for us and is doing, we should strive our best to keep our level of consciousness always at the highest we are capable of.

If we do that, there is a standing sanction from her that every wish, at the height of our consciousness, shall be fulfilled. Our responsibility is to keep ourselves at the zenith possible to us.

She is fully aware of the difficulties, of the nature of the trials, that have to be faced in Auroville. But her stress is on development of consciousness and she sees everything in terms of that. For her, outer difficulties are a faithful reflection of the inner obstructions put up by individuals living here.

About thirteen years ago she once explained to me that as long as inmates of the ashram were solely devoted to yogic pursuits, had their mind fixed on the spiritual goal, she had absolutely no difficulty regarding finance. She had actually more than what was needed and things used to go absolutely smoothly.

It was only when more people started coming — when she had to admit more numbers as a result of the second World War and the influx of refugees from Eastern India — that a certain dilution took place. Ordinary desires and motive-forces entered the atmosphere. And what is more important, wastage started. Since then the flow of money and resources has been impeded, and the acute difficulty of money is an everyday affair.

I wrote to Mother and asked, "Why is it, that in every household outside, anybody praying to you, anybody writing to you of financial difficulties, gets relief. Within a month we get their next letter saying that the help has reached them; their conditions have improved. Then why is it that under your very physical presence we are having these financial stringencies?"

Mother said, "I am helpless. This is governed more by the atmosphere, by the kind of thoughts and emotions that are current in the atmosphere. They attract or they repel money." And wastage is a primary thing which repels the inflow of money-power.

Whether there is wastage in Auroville is for you to see. I am not competent to say because I do not stay here. If each one of you takes steps to eliminate wastage in the area where you have a say, that is the way towards the elimination of general wastage and toward encouragement, invocation, of the necessary resources for the speedier building of Auroville.

Perhaps having said all this I should conclude with an apposite story. One day a young boy brought up this topic during the question hour at the playground when Mother was holding a class. "Mother", he said, "so much wastage is going on in the ashram. Why are you allowing it in the departments and elsewhere?" Mother became serious and said "The wastage of money and materials doesn't touch me so much as the wastage of spiritual energy that is going on. It is that which is depressing."

So that also is a point to ponder. How much spiritual wastage is going on in each one of us, through each one of us in moments of unconsciousness, or half-consciousness or wilful indulgence.

6

Release from Subjection to the Body, Heart and Mind

At the close of our discussion on the subject of release from subjection to the physical body, we made an observation that we had to deal with *prana*, that is the life-force, as it acts on the mind and the heart. We will now discuss in certain detail the exact process of this operation of the life-forces on the heart and mind, and the method that is adopted in the yoga of knowledge for releasing oneself from this subjection.

It is the business of the life-force, in this world, to move and to act. It always insists upon darting forward, — in the movement of the senses, in the movement of the thought,— seizing an object and reporting it to the intelligence. But this life-force that acts as a channel, as a link between ourselves and the things outside of us, is not a pure channel. It is mixed with desire, impelled by desire and its report is tainted with desire. Rarely does the life-force bring back the contact precisely in the form in which it is presented. If it suits its desire-impulse, there is the reaction of like, of preference. If it does not, if it conflicts with it, the reaction is one of dislike. This duality of like and dislike, pleasure and pain, is the contribution of the desire-infected life-force to the situation. A seeker of the yoga of knowledge has necessarily to take account of this feature of the working of the life-force.

There is, first, the mind of the senses, the sensational mind, thereafter, the emotional mind and thereafter the thought mind. Now all these three are mixed in their operation with the workings of the life-force. The sense activity is completely vitiated by the preferences, the likings, the repulsions and the attractions of the desire-led life-force. Similarly, the emotional mind — what we call the heart, presided over by the emotional mind — is likewise interfered with by desires. Likings, attachments, rebuffs, repulsions — all these based upon a basic desire misreport the situation. And this life-being on the wings of the life-force, we mistake for the soul.

Actually, what we thus call the soul is not the soul at all; it is what Sri Aurobindo calls the "desire-soul". The desire mind bases itself upon the soul-projection in nature, and masquerades as the true soul. That is at the root of ninety percent of the unhappiness in the human world. Similarly in the thought mind whether the thought mind is conscious of it or not, the bias imparted by the desire mind perverts the judgement of the thought mind, inclines it to preferences, choosings and gives what we may generally call a biased view of everything.

These three pollutions, the pollutions by the desire-soul of the sense-mind, the emotional mind and the thought mind, are to be first remedied. And how are we to remedy them? The process is the same with all — detachment. The being, the *purusha*, has first to detach itself from involvement, take up a witness position, and say to itself, "I am not this life-force, I am not this desire mind, I am not even this sense mentality, this emotional mentality, this thought operation. They are the specialised workings of nature, on particular planes, which are twisted by the desire-dominated life-force."

Once the mind learns this habit of what the Mother calls "standing back" and refusing its complete identification with nature movements, a certain gulf is created. No doubt the gulf is again overwhelmed in the avalanche of the movements of nature, of desires, passions and seekings of the desire soul, still, when man becomes an awakened being, a conscious being, he can re-exert his will to disengage himself from this helpless involvement and effect a kind of bifurcation, in time, between his self and the operations of nature. So done, the mind comes to a position when it looks upon itself as the central being, the mental *purusha*, on whom everything else depends.

But beware. Even this is a projection of the ego in the mind. As we have observed, the ego has any number of avatars. It masquerades, it hides behind many specious pleas, and the fact that this ego-point, this ego, is senior in time to our mental being, our vital being and the physical being gives it a certain advantage. For, as you know, the ego is the first centralising point formed by nature in order to give a certain fixity in the flux of life. Before the ego forms, it is only a flow of life, a flow of mentality. When nature laboriously, industriously erects, fashions a point around which it organises the activity, the flow of experience, the ego-entity is formed. In the course of evolution this entity grows into a personality.

This ego has got such a powerful hold that even when by a rigorous process of disengagement, non-identification, one releases oneself from the activity of the ego, the egoity, the spirit of the ego remains. Men who have got release from the formulated activity of ego flatter themselves into the belief that they have been liberated but actually they launch into a career of a magnified ego, a magniloquent career of egoity. For the spirit of the ego sticks. And as long as the ego or egoity is strong the psychic being can never emerge. Even a ray of the psychic being — when it gets through — is captured by the ego which gives it its own coating and claims for itself a further lease of life.

The prescription for this malady of the ego in the traditional yoga of knowledge is to affirm to oneself thus: "I am not this personality, I am not this ego"; negatively to negate identification with the ego and positively to affirm one's identity, at the core, with the Reality. The Reality —

which reality? There is a reality within; there is a reality without; there is a reality beyond. The traditional yoga of knowledge points to that essence of Reality within oneself, that point in the core of the heart whence all derives, which waits for one's approach, behind a hundred veils. That it calls the self, which is called the Monad in Western philosophy.

This self, this *jiva* as it is termed in Sanskrit, what we may call the being, the real being, is associated with nature but is not a creature of nature. Actually, it is a projection of the Supreme Self that sustains, that presides over the universe. Projected in the individual scheme it is the self, the individual self. And what we call nature is, on a certain level, its own power. On a lower level we call this nature *prakriti*; on a higher level we call it puissance, power, *shakti*. So in the original status, the self, the *jiva*, the being, is the master, but we do not realise that poise of mastery immediately.

In the yoga of which we are speaking, the process begins by quieting the restless movement of the mind and the agitation of the vital, the life-force, so that in the calm, in the silence that ensues in the being, some reflection of the inner self may be experienced. True, periods of this experience are clouded over again and again when we descend back into the life of nature. But each time there is this delving within we move on, if I may say so, at least a centimeter further. And whatever may be the appearance, though we may think we have come back to the same old movements of nature, it is not so in fact. We are one step removed from the old involvement.

First the witness, then the silence, then the reflection; thereafter, a continuous remembrance of what has been experienced. Recalling, visualising in the mind, re-experiencing in the consciousness the same movement of that radical experience brings about an enlargement of that experience. And so, one progresses more and more inwards till there is a sudden snapping of the knots of the desire-soul and one lands in the lap of the inner monarch. That is only the first step, though a capital one.

After realising this inner Divine, the next step, according to the yoga of knowledge, is to realise that this Reality, this irreducible Reality within, is none other than the Absolute, than the Brahman. The identity is always there behind, behind nature. The process is to relax, to get back, and find the link between one's reality, one's self and the Supreme, the Absolute, the Brahman.

There are differences in belief among philosophers, people who have got spiritual realisations, as to the nature of this what they call the 'ultimate experience'. Whether the reality that is my self completely merges in the Supreme Reality and is no more, or it realises its identity but continues its distinct individuality against the background of the Absolute Reality, are matters to be discussed in philosophical debates, but have no relevance to us. For we are concerned with the practical dynamics of the situation, and both Sri Aurobindo and the Mother have pointed out that it is not only possible, but inevitable, as a result of an integral approach and an integral practice, that the individual reality can at some level feel one with the Supreme, and simultaneously, in another poise, on another level, it can maintain a certain relation of intimacy, of mutuality with the Absolute. It is possible to realise both the experiences.

So far regarding the contribution, or the vision, of the traditional yoga of knowledge. To the seeker of the integral yoga, however, this is not enough. It is not enough for him to realise his own divinity, and either merge in the Supreme Divinity, or have personal relations with it. His perception, his realisation of the divinity within is not complete unless he realises the existence of the same divinity in others. Till he comes out of the confines of his being, extends his consciousness, and embraces the whole universe in the endless arms of his consciousness, his realisation on earth is not complete. It is only as his mind breaks its frontiers of thought and his heart opens its gates and receives contacts from outside without restriction, without reacting, without hesitation, without repulsion, but with a wide compassion and love, that the second step of the yoga nears completion. In a side observation, Sri Aurobindo makes a pertinent remark on how what we call, what generally passes for compassion and is expressed in terms of pity, helping others, is not really born in most cases out of genuine love, out of genuine identification with others, but is a camouflaged regard for one's own feelings. One cannot stand the sight of the suffering of others; there is a revulsion, the nervous being is unable to stand the sight. And, to prevent that, to save oneself from that situation, one goes to help.

Now, this kind of help based upon self-regard has no spiritual value. A spiritual value ensues only when one feels the pain of another in the being, and as a result something appeals to that part which is a reservoir of love, and compassion, and there is an outflow of the sea of love and compassion. That is spiritual help.

It is inevitable in the second step — what is called the cosmic realisation, the realisation of the Cosmic Self that the individual self has to realise its identity with the Cosmic Self. Even then the journey is not over; the individual self and the Cosmic Self are both projections, in creation, of a Transcendent Self which always exceeds these two formations of the Self. It is certainly not *beyond* in the sense of having no relations with the earth as in Buddhist philosophy, nor as in the Adwaita philosophy of Shankara, where the Absolute is conceived as something totally transcendent of this universe and the individual and when one realises it all sinks into negation, all looks like a figment of an imagination or a dream. That is not the truth, though certain experiences give an appearance of truth to it. The Reality is no doubt transcendent, but it is an Absolute which contains the relative.

The relative has not come out of nothing, the relative has come out of the bosom of the Absolute. So even while exceeding it, even while transcending it, the relation continues. All the three terms of the Reality, — the Transcendental, the Universal or the Cosmic, the Individual — all these three are real as related to this manifestation and in the measure in which one releases oneself from the subjection to the body, the subjection to the ego-sense in the life-force, in the mind and in the heart, one begins to experience the truth of this triple Reality of existence.

Any questions?

Is the physical mind the same as the sense mind, the thought mind? What are the four minds spoken of here?

The classifications of the mind differ according to the standpoint accepted. The classification of which I spoke — the sense mind, the emotive mind and the thought mind etc. — is of the ancient Indian system, which is followed in the traditional system of knowledge. Sri Aurobindo's classification is of the physical mind, the vital mind, the reasoning mind, then the higher mind, the illumined mind, and so on. There is a certain overlapping. Though, as you said, the physical mind can be broadly equated with the sense mind, since it depends entirely on the activity of the senses, the physical mind also has its thought content.

I remember how once it was in 1940 or 41 when there was a criticism about some book of Sri Aurobindo's by a professor in Calcutta and I had replied to it, Sri Aurobindo had practically summarised a paragraph of mine in one sentence. He wrote in the margin, *"The physical mind also thinks."*

So it has a thinking activity; the thinking activity does not belong to the thought mind alone. The vital mind also thinks, but as Mother says, it thinks very cunningly (laughter). In philosophical parlance, you can call that the thought mind which moves in the realm of ideas, to which thinking is more important than anything else. Nothing is true to it unless it is thought out. The dominating force is reason.

It is only when man realises the limitations of the thought mind that he opens to the realms above the mind. Though for most, the problem doesn't arise, because in them even the thought mind is not active. They mostly live in the physical mind and the vital mind. And in yoga, when they are told to silence the mind it is these layers, the physical and vital that are to be quieted, surrendered to the action of the higher force. So the confusing and doubting activity of the thought mind does not enter into many people who are undeveloped. Actually it is yogically an advantage not to have an active thought mind (laughter).

Is there a psychic mind or a subtle mind?

Not really but that part of the mind which is under the influence of the psychic, receives the psychic rays and influence and reacts from that basis may be described as the psychic mind. Though the position proper of the psychic is not in the mind but in the heart, its influence may spread into the mind. For instance, when the psychic perception is active we may think that our mind is perceiving, but it is this psychic perception that reflects itself in the mental discrimination. The impulse is from the psychic.

Then when Sri Aurobindo speaks of receiving messages and illumination from the higher light does he mean the psychic?

No, not the psychic. The mind, as far as it is developed, falls silent. And when it is silent and does not interfere, then the messages that come down from above or rise up from below are received here in the mind. The mind can receive messages from the heart, that is the psychic, as also from the Spirit above. Man being what he is, the mind is the receiving center.

When one opens to inspiration, does his nature change?

Often, it acts through the vital mind and after the

inspiration is over the man continues to be an ordinary man. If the being had developed, if the mind, the vital were in tune, purified, then such infusion, descent of inspiration, should make a tremendous difference in the consciousness of the person. When it does not, it means that only a part has been instrumentalised — as with some painters. They are wonderful when they are in the painting mood, when they are doing their work. Mother has so often spoken of certain people, — how marvellous they were when they were composing music, when they were painting. But afterwards, when the inspiration stopped, they turned out to be very ordinary. It is only when there is a certain kind of integration where there is at least a working unification of the being around the developed part, that what is received in the developed part can have a powerful effect on the whole. That calls for yoga.

Can one share the experiences of another and by so doing help them?

Unless one is truly detached, one can't share the experience of another. If one is involved, it is only a superficial, sense contact. My sharing of your pain doesn't help you in any way. Only when I am detached, am I able to take, consciously, your pain and lessen your burden. It is a conscious taking, not a helpless subjection, which comes by detachment.

By detachment you separate yourself, you rise above nature and you command the situation. Just as a physical mother, when she sees her child suffering, picks it up, soothes it, and restores it to normalcy, similarly when a yogin sympathises with a sufferer his consciousness takes on the man's burden to the extent that is permitted by his *karma*, and in the very process of taking it on consciously, which he is able to do because he is detached, the other person gets relief.

I distinctly remember how when I was about 13 or 14, I used to get a burning sensation in my ears and my ears used to get red. No doctor could help, nobody knew what to do. But it happened many times that I never had that burning sensation as long as my guru was with me in the same room. I was not aware of this until suddenly somebody remarked that my guru's ears were red and hot. He had taken on my suffering. I speak from personal experience. If he had had no detachment, in spite of his sympathy he could not have relieved me of that pain.

I am speaking only of physical pain. There are many kinds of pain: physical pain, psychological pain, spiritual pain. Indian tradition speaks of three kinds of suffering.

One cannot enlarge one's consciousness, one cannot embrace others in one's consciousness unless one first attains a degree of detachment from nature. Otherwise the consciousness is bound to the individual nature.

But how can one concentrate on one point and yet open both inwardly and upwardly?

Actually, the psychic has been compared to a flame, to a point of light. It is the fine end of the spirit in one's body. So when you contact the psychic there is an automatic link with the spirit, of which it is a projection in evolution. It is the spirit that stands aloof that we call the Central Being; it is the same spirit, when projected in evolving nature, in evolution, that starts as a point and develops into an entity. That entity develops into a being and that being develops into a personality. So when you contact the psychic, when you concentrate upon the psychic there is an immediate response from the spirit. One need not shift the center of concentration; one has to allow it to develop. There one has to be only an observer. The operation of concentration should be left to itself to move here or there. Whatever it is, we have not to interfere with our mind. There there is not this dimension of up and below; it is our mind that translates this happening in terms of vertical and horizontal because we are used to this space formula.

There are stories — actual renderings from life — where

it is told that when they are in that state people have wondered whether the soul is in the body or the body is in the soul. And Sri Aurobindo had even narrated a story from one of the scriptures about a disciple wondering whether the elephant was on the rider or the rider on the elephant. The whole thing gets topsy-turvy from our standpoint until the perception settles sufficiently, plastically. Then we know there is neither above nor below; all is one. It depends upon the angle from which we see, the poise from which we experience.

Is that what Mother means in her message 'when you are conscious of the whole world at the same time, then you can become conscious of the Divine'?

Yes. When the physical barriers of space are broken down there is one psychological space in which we are conscious of anything happening anywhere if we want to know. That is the attainment of the Universal Consciousness. It is not that we are all the time conscious of what is happening everywhere, but when we want to know we have only to will it and we know it. For instance if I want I can know what is going on in your mind or what is happening at the moment in the United States — because there there is no physical distance.

In dreams, for instance, — it gives some idea — when we are sleeping we cover the whole world. We travel anywhere we like, we meet many people — and that experience, at the time it takes place, is real. The order of experience is different, but the experience is real, nonetheless. The senses that are active in the dream state respond in the same way as the physical senses do when in the waking condition. So that shows the possibility of transcending the barriers of physical space and division.

When and how can the knots be snapped?

The final snapping is always preceded by a lot of loosening — a conscious, willed loosening by oneself or a loosening by a series of shocks, unwelcome experiences which hammer and loosen the tangled webs. But the final release comes from a sudden snapping. The Upanishad speaks of the knots of the heart snapping by an act of Grace; it does not happen by human effort. That final release from the knot is beyond human capacity because in a sense it came into being before one was born. It has been fashioned by Nature, and it is a higher nature, a stroke of Grace that alone can snap it. Different mystic traditions give different imageries. When the final knot snaps, the revelations of the inner Divine is a fact and the possibility of realising the universal Divine is near, the door is open to the ascent above.

It is possible to go into the beyond leaving the heart knot where it is. In the traditional methods they just leave the whole system, the body, the personality as it is and hook on to the mind. First they have a certain mental experience, mental realisation and then cutting off connections with the whole being, they disappear into the Absolute — maybe the silence of Buddha or the Bliss of Shankara. That they can do because they do not insist upon carrying the whole being where they go. They ignore it; it has not helped anybody.

Can this happen when the ego is still active?

It can't happen. After all, the ego is not a real person; it is a shadow. It is a shadow of the true person, and the shadow exists as long as that certain perverse knot continues, giving it a chance to continue. Once that is snapped, the true being emerges in its light, without the shadow. The gods, it is said in the Puranas, have no shadow. They don't sleep, their eyes don't wink, they carry no shadow.

I suppose one has to have a cosmic realisation before one can be conscious of the Divine?

No, one can be conscious of the Divine even without the cosmic realisation. To be conscious of the Divine is one thing; to realise the Divine is another; to embody and manifest the Divine is still another. One is conscious at a point. One lives it, lives the Divine on a certain plane of living to begin with — that has to be extended. When this realisation of the Divine, this Divine consciousness is organised, made to occupy the whole of the being, including the body, then one can say that one embodies the Divine Consciousness. It is a far cry from being conscious of the Divine to be able to embody the Divine.

7

The Realisation of the Cosmic Self

The island ego joined its continent.

This was the note on which we concluded last time. It is a famous line from Sri Aurobindo's *Savitri,* describing the dissolution of the ego-personality of Aswapathy, but not the annihilation of his personality. It says it joined its continent; his consciousness joins — not merges, but joins — the larger consciousness of which it is really a part. And that is our subject this evening — in what way does one proceed, after certain radical steps have been taken, for the dissolution of the ego.

When one withdraws from the external life of the body, life and mind and turns one's preoccupation inward in search of the Self, gradually a certain detachment is effected from the external life activity. And with appropriate discipline and sustained effort, one arrives ultimately at the realisation of identity with one's true self. That is the end in many of lines of spiritual tradition. Of course, for us it is only a step, though a capital step, leading to other, further steps.

When one arrives at identity with the self, one realises that what one thought to be one's real life — the external life — is not the true life, for one's true life begins with the attainment of identity with the self. But another question arises: what shall be the relation between the self now realised and the life of the mind, the life-force and the body that one has left behind? There is always a tendency to regard this life that one has left behind as something inferior, transitory, what is called a "passing show" on the bosom of the silent, immutable Self. Even as one makes the mistake while engrossed in the worldly life, of considering the concept of the Self, the concept of the soul as something fanciful, something superstitious, irrational, similarly when one arrives in the domain of the Self proper, there is this tendency to pay back the compliment, to regard the usual life, the mundane life as it is as fanciful, false, dispensable. But for the seeker of the Integral Path that option is not open simply because it is baseless.

The position we start with is that the Spirit, the Self, and the material world, are two rungs of one gradation: the Spirit in its status at the top, the evolving life at the bottom, on earth, but with a constant relation between them. One has to find this relation in the Self; the relation between the transcendent Self, and the world is to be found in the depths of the Self where all converge. If it is true, if it is open to experience and realisation that the divine Self can be realised in oneself, can be perceived and experienced around oneself and contacted beyond this world, beyond both the universe and the individual, man being capable of identification in his essence with the Divine, should also be able to reproduce this relation, to share in the same experience. And one of the oldest of the Indian Upanishads affirms that not only can it be so, but it has to be so.

The perspective that this tradition of ancient thought gives is to regard all things, all forms, all beings in the Self. Not only that but also the Self itself in the forms and the Self as the forms. An equally old Upanishad puts it graphically. It says, "He desired, when he was alone, to be the Many, to manifest, and out of his own being he projected this creation of forms and movements." He was not satisfied with creating and releasing the world; creating, he entered into it. He entered, not merely in a general way in the creation, but individually, in each form, he entered. He is the indweller in each one; he creates, he enters and he dwells. All the three capital steps have been described graphically in the Upanishads. It says, "The spirit desired of old, 'I would be manifold for the birth of peoples'; therefore he concentrated all of himself in thought and by the force of his brooding he created all this universe, all whatsoever exists. Now, when he had brought it forth, he entered into that he had created. Entering, he became the 'is here' and the 'may be there'; he became that which is defined and that which has no feature; he became this housed thing and that houseless; he became knowledge and he became ignorance; he became Truth, he became Falsehood. He became all Truth, even whatsoever here exists, therefore they say of him that he is Truth."

This is the broad perspective that the seeker of the way of knowledge must always have. First, he envisages this universe not as a creation of a power of illusion, of a power of falsehood, of an inferior origin but as a deliberate creation, a self-projection of the Eternal. The Infinite projects the finite out of its bosom. The finite is as much real as the Infinite from which it emerges. Essentially the degree of reality is the same, but in manifesting, in creating, in projecting out of itself, the Infinite, the Eternal does not become subject to what it creates. It is not subject to time and space which are but circumstances contained in its projection. All movements, all circumstances and conditions are subsequent to the act of creation. Having created, the Eternal continues to be what it is. It is free: When the ancient seers say,'it is not this', 'it is not that', it does not mean that it is different from the Eternal, that it is not the Eternal. It simply means that the Eternal, the Infinite is not exhausted by it. The Eternal is not completely held or contained in any of its creatures, but on that account the fact that each form, each creature derives directly from the Reality cannot be denied.

So this is the first realisation — first, to believe mentally, second, to feel in the heart — that must be realised in day-to-day life that this spectacular world, this creation, this universe is a projection, a purposive creation of the Lord. He it is who has become the many. If one stays in that realisation alone, one feels the whole movement of the world, together with all the living creatures and beings passing like so many figures, images, shadows, and in its haste to come to a conclusion, the human mind decides that the world consists of images and figures, figments of some colossal imagination passing on the surface of the ineffable, white pure Self. That is an exaggeration.

If we persist in our quest for the truth, we become aware that the Divine Reality we have realised is not only in the depths or on the heights of our own being, but it is also to be found in the depths and on the heights of other beings. He who dwells in me dwells equally in my neighbour, in another; also, not only it dwells in human forms, but in all forms. This truth is at the basis of the unity of creation. No doubt we are separated by fragmentation in form, by division in consciousness consequent on the birth of egoism, but at a certain level there is the oneness. And that oneness is of the Divine Self, which is equally spread out, and if I want to realise my unity with others, with the rest of the world, that true unity can be realised only on that basis where my Self and the Self of others meet. There is, no doubt, only one Self, but it has posited itself at innumerable centres. It is at the level of the Self that one breathes a natural oneness.

Till then, till the spiritual realisation of the Self in all, the common Self between me and you is realised, all else is talk — may be preparatory talk to build up the climate, to accustom the mind so that the whole being is readied to receive the truth when it dawns. Unless this realisation and attainment are true on our soul level, they remain mere acquirements of mental knowledge.

Well, the second truth leads to the third. It is not enough to have relations with other forms, with other creatures, with the world at large if the Divine is there only as an indweller in each form. What about the form of the self? What about the structure? The true spiritual knowledge says that even the forms — everything — are the Divine Self. All in the Self, the Self in the all, all *as* the Self. The two earlier truths are incomplete without this culminating truth of the Self as the All.

This is the general truth, but how does one realise it oneself? It is by identifying oneself, in the soul, with the manifesting Divine. The Divine, the sole Being, in its aspect of manifesting, is throwing itself out into a multiple becoming. By identifying myself with my soul, I can also experience this movement of my being flowing into so many becomings.

There are a number of disciplines that are used to train the mind to participate in this spiritual attainment. The Upanishad speaks of concentration and meditation using the image of the ether — not this gross ether but the supreme, the highest ether, from which all creation emerges. Of course, the physical sky, the physical ether, being part of the supreme Ether, can be taken as a helpful imagery. Just as ether envelops all, yet constitutes all and contains all, the spirit too envelops all, enters all and holds all in itself. This constant image — the spirit, like the ether is everywhere — promotes a certain freedom for the mind from its petty involvement in local movements. The mind gets disinvolved, gets purified, with this constant affirmation of the freedom of the spirit, of the freedom of which one is capable by growing in the spirit and yet retaining the true relation that is possible with the universe.

The first step, indeed, is gradually to acquire control and finally eliminate the ego. Second, the mental horizon must be slowly expanded. One starts with an intellectual belief, no doubt, but one translates it, to the extent it is possible, in day-to-day life into practice. Similarly, the life emotions — sympathies, understandings, love, compassion — instead of being confined to our own interest and to the interest of those with whom we are closely identified, by whatever ties, are allowed a free scope, and the body itself is taught not to regard itself as a separate entity, but as a part dependent upon the universal Matter, drawing sustenance from the universe. It is impressed upon the life-force that it is but one wave of the ocean of Life around, and the mind understands that it is but one chamber, one fragment of the universal Mind and all its thoughts are rays that go out and emerge — and immerge — in the universal Light around. These are certain lines of proceeding towards the exceeding of the personal, limited, individual consciousness and expanding, enlarging, breaking out into the larger consciousness which is variously called the Universal Consciousness, the Cosmic Consciousness.

Many have had this perception that once man exceeds his present mental, limited, ego-based consciousness and enters into the realm of the universal consciousness, things undergo a radical change. There is a famous Canadian doctor, who had a strong experience of this cosmic consciousness all of a sudden, and what he writes, after affirming that experience in himself, after undergoing the changes that are inevitable after the experience, is interesting. He says:

> In contact with the flux of cosmic consciousness, all religions known and named today, will be melted down. The human soul will be revolutionised. Religion will absolutely dominate the race. (He means by religion spirituality.) It will not be in sacred books nor in the mouths of priests. It will not teach of future immortality nor future glories, for immortality and all glory exists in the here and now. The evidence of immortality will live in every heart, as sight in every eye. Doubt of God and of eternal life will be impossible, as is now doubt of existence. Churches, priests, forms, creeds, prayers — all agents, all intermediaries between the individual

> man and God will be permanently replaced by direct, unmistakable intercourse. Each soul will feel and know itself to be immortal, will feel and know that the entire universe, with all its good and with all its beauty, is for it and belongs to it forever. The world peopled by men possessing cosmic consciousness will be as far removed from the world today as this from the world as it was before the advent of self-consciousness. This new race is in the act of being born from us, and in the near future will occupy and possess the earth.

. . . A most prophetic announcement made *at least four* decades ago.

This stage of realising the cosmic consciousness, or at any rate, of experiencing oneness with all, having a flow of love for all (which is one of the results of opening to the cosmic consciousness), is an indispensable step for what the Mother calls 'transformation'. It is a must for everyone who hopes to belong to the new age. Particularly for those who are working and striving for the new consciousness this experience, this realisation, or at least an opening to the universal or cosmic consciousness is the first important step to be worked out.

I was speaking to someone regarding what exactly is implied when a person is admitted either into the Ashram or into Auroville. There is a facile tendency to feel that once one is admitted or made a member of either Auroville or the Ashram, one has qualified, one has got the requirement to be a member of the new race. But it is not so. Both Sri Aurobindo and the Mother have repeatedly said that all that it means is that a possibility is seen in the individual concerned; his evolution has arrived at a stage when that possibility of transcending the old and emerging into the new appears in the soul. Once the possibility is seen, the Mother gives a chance to the person to build upon it, to actualise that possibility. The opportunity is given, the field is opened, the grace is sanctioned. The rest is left to the individual — to put in his personal effort, to take advantage of the opportunities given to him, and to develop himself in the mould of the ideal placed before him.

This is one point I had to make clear because I have been repeatedly asked, "Why I am asked to go away? If Mother did not consider me fit, why did she allow me to come?" This is the answer — she saw a possibility; you walked back upon it.

Questions and Answers

You had some questions to ask about mind?

Yes, the four minds . . .

There are not really four minds, but many more . . .

Infinite, is it?

Not that. Broadly speaking, the mind is that part of our nature which thinks, which cognizes, which deals in ideas. But this mind has so many layers. That mind which is always concerned with physical things, attending to physical comforts, dealing in physical movements, its whole attention riveted on physical creature comforts, depends only on physical data to think, to formulate — that is called the physical mind.

That part of the mind which is involved in the movements of emotions, desires, ambitions — justifying them, giving them a colour of rational movements, expressing them in terms of thought — that is called the vital mind. The mind which deals on the data of senses — each time an object comes before them the senses rush to make an impact, give the report — collects all these reports (mostly, as Mother says, false reports) coordinates them and builds up its own insecure, unsound knowledge — that is called the sense mind.

Above the sense mind there is the reasoning mind which reasons — this is so, that is so — whether the reason is correct or not is a different matter; but it reasons even in a vacuum. Above the reasoning mind is the thought mind, where the mind moves in the dimensions of thinking — it's not so much concerned with practical matters; above the thought mind is the ideative mind of pure ideas. Here ideas have not yet taken the form of thoughts. Broad principles, broad ideative movements — they are the ideative mind.

Above these ranges of the intellectual mind are the ranges of the spiritual mind, of which what Sri Aurobindo calls the higher mind is the lowest rung. Above the higher mind is the illumined mind; above the illumined mind is the intuitive mind; above the intuitive is the overmind and above the overmind is the supermind.

The body itself has a small mind. That is, the projection of the physical part in the mental layers — it is called the physical mind. Even when our mind is otherwise occupied, the body thinks; for example the leg automatically draws back if there is danger. So there is a sort of mechanical mind in which the summit of the physical projects into the region of the mind. This is the body mind.

Similarly, if there is a part of the mind involved in the vital, there is a part of the vital which projects into the mental. That is called the mental vital; the vital being, the vital part with a mental colouring.

Now to distinguish the vital mind and the mental vital you must note the word that ends the phrase, for that gives the clue. "Vital mind" — that means the vital part of the mind; here mind is the main thing. So with "mental vital" here the vital is the main thing; the mental is that part of the vital which has a mental nature, which has its own way of thinking, of planning.

Naturally, these divisions in Sri Aurobindo's philosophy don't exactly tally with those made by philosophers and thinkers in Europe. What they call the unconscious, the subconscious, is quite different. What they call the unconscious is what we call the subliminal — that part which is behind the external, waking intelligence of which we are normally not cognizant. The larger mind, the larger vital, the larger physical, touching the universal mind, the universal life and the universal matter — that is the subliminal. The subliminal ranges from top to toe. The whole is simply called the unconscious by certain philosophers in Europe now in fashion, simply because we are not conscious of it. It is conscious in its own way, perhaps more intensified, with a larger range. I do not know what the subliminal means to the Western philosophers in Europe like Freud, but to us what the subliminal means is what I have just said. Certainly it is not unconscious.

After the conscious level there follows the subconscious — subconscious means the half-conscious. Below the subconscious is the unconscious where we are not at all conscious. But even in that domain of unconsciousness, there is a ray of consciousness which is not active on the surface. When even that ray is congealed, becomes a block, that is the inconscience, practically a total nescience. If you delve deep into the inconscient, you will find some throb of what develops, ultimately, into consciousness.

The Mother has said that it is to re-vivify this state of nescience that the Grace descended in the form of a ray of consciousness and light and started the return journey of the soul.

In the meeting before the last one you were discussing the states of sleep and dream. You said that they are always present whether we are walking around. If one is trying to be conscious of this, and one is conscious when one is dreaming or just walking around, is there something further one can do, because it seems as though those things have a tremendous effect on the whole nervous system.

When you go further than being just conscious of being in a dream, the dream stops, the dream consciousness is converted into the waking consciousness.

What if one has been changing one's dreams?

That is, you assert your will and change the happening

in the dream — is that what you mean?

Yes.

It is an interesting exercise. It means some things are going on and you are consciously participating in the events on the subtler planes. They can have an indicatory value, a significance which can translate itself in day-to day life. But, to dwell too much in dream experiences leads to a certain subjectivism and one's hold on the waking condition weakens.

It is always advisable to increase the range of the waking consciousness, to bring even in sleep and dream the control of the will of the waking consciousness. Instead of dwelling longer and longer in those areas, the sleep element, the dream element must be shortened as much as possible. Because our whole aim is to increase the content of consciousness, expand the range of consciousness. The rest, the peace, the recuperation that the body needs is being constantly and incessantly made available to it when one part dwells in peace. When you are able to bifurcate your being and consciousness — the frontal part participating in work, and the other not participating but open to Peace and Silence —simultaneously, the process of recuperation goes on, and you need sleep less and less. That is why one of the signs of the progress of yoga is that one begins to need less food, less sleep, less company.

Of course, there are periods, particularly in lines of meditation, where at times one is obliged to sleep longer because the consciousness withdraws, indraws itself. And whether in trance of meditation or what appears to be sleep, some work is going on inside. But these are periods of yogic working, not sleep in the sense in which an average man takes it to be.

Till quite recently the Mother never had a bed. She used to always recline on a chair. Just when you go up to her room, on the first floor, before you turn to the small staircase leading upstairs, there is a cushioned seat; it has a footrest, and that was the place where she used to rest. In the morning she would receive us there to transact business but at night there was a fan there (normally she is averse to fans but somehow it is there) and that was all. She never slept; she never had a pillow. It is only recently that, under the advice and insistence of medical doctors, she has agreed to have a regular bed, though even when she is not well she spends most of the time in the chair.

There have been others also who sleep very nominally. There is a saying in Sanskrit that three types of people don't have sleep during nights: a *yogi*, a *rogi* — who is sick and diseased —, a *bhogi* — who enjoys himself in the sensual way. It is a saying which sums up quite a philosophy.

Recently we heard that the Mother has given a very wonderful name for one of the Auroville children - she called him 'Auromaharshi'. When she gives a name does she see a tendency in the child and names it according to something that is present or does she give something for the child's development?

When the thing is brought before her — either a letter or a report — when the thing is presented, immediately she sees something, answering to the situation, the truth that is trying to express itself. You take a picture of a child and you ask for a name. Immediately she knows what is the truth behind it, she gives that name.

Similarly with children; she sees what is trying to manifest there. Possibly it must be somebody — a maharshi, you say, some great sage who has chosen to embody himself and pursue his quest. He has come for transformation, to belong to the new race; that way, she has seen a number of particular souls who have come. She doesn't always speak but she has been doing that for a number of years, even before Auroville started, with children who have been joining the Ashram. She knows who they are. And there are one or two who died during Mother's present life and have come where Mother is here now. They were with Mother before, in this present life, and they died and now they have taken birth here.

Does she call people at any time?

She doesn't call them, but in answer to their own aspiration, in conformity with the work assigned to them by the Supreme, these souls come. In fact, a host of them, we are told, are waiting in the subtle-physical world for conditions to be ready for a supramental birth; they do not care very much to have the animal type of birth and they are waiting for the new processes to be perfected when they will all project themselves on earth. Whether we will be there alive or not I do not know (laughter).

It may be tomorrow, it may be a hundred years hence, we can't say. The conception of time is different on those planes.

Is it this same vision of recognition that enables Mother to refuse or accept Aurovillians?

Not always, not always. She doesn't go so deep. She once explained that she doesn't decide anything without a sign from within. There are people who she feels have come for this work. When she sees them, sees their picture if they are of the category that has come to participate in this life, she doesn't consider anything else — their money, their background, nothing — she straight away admits them. But there are people who are not of that type, who are not ready, but who have a possibility of getting ready and there she considers other factors — whether the person can maintain himself, whether the person has certain capacities to serve etc. The secondary considerations come when the category is different. In some she feels, she doesn't go beyond that feeling. In some she sees. But where she concentrates, she always knows. She does not concentrate always, due to so many factors — people around her talking too much, intervening, or lack of time etc. That is where as I put it the luck of the person comes in.

Is there also a consideration of the work to be done, at this time for example, the movement to bring India and America closer together. Are there some who can serve in that capacity at this time, so that their place is there rather than here?

She thinks in terms of the whole universe, not in terms of countries. In her vision the whole Globe is one. These things are usually proposed and then permitted or sanctioned. Ultimately she works on her plane. We can support that work, become instruments of her working, to the extent that we develop our consciousness, be in tune with hers. We need not develop to that height, but at least we can be in tune; those who do so are her real instruments. The real work is done on the plane of consciousness; the results are seen as they germinate on the physical level afterwards. Any physical instruments may come in at that time. But the real work is done earlier.

Certainly America is drawing closer. But the work has been done in 1939 — ever since the *Life Divine* appeared and the first copy went to America, and was received there — somehow it was in Sri Aurobindo's consciousness that this new, young continent has a big part to play in the new creation. Even recently the Mother said that there is much wealth waiting in America to serve in Auroville. If it has not found its way, it is due to certain lacunae here such as want of the proper attitude, receptivity etc.

So not only Europe, America, but other countries too have all got to play their part. And they have, I believe, begun to do it. Only those who embody a developed consciousness, a spiritual consciousness, something of the new consciousness, will be able to make a lasting and radical impact on the leaders of thought and life in other countries. Merely to talk, to write, is not enough. There are plenty of clever writers, impressive speakers who are already doing it, but that has not clicked. One has to carry this flame so that those who hear catch it, those who hear find a new dimension opened in their being. It is that that is more important.

It is the minds that have to be drawn, it is the men that have to be drawn; not so much money or machinery.

8

The Modes of the Self

We have come to the stage in our study in *The Synthesis of Yoga* where, I believe, it will be useful to have a certain clarification of the terms that we will be using rather frequently from now on.

I thought of this after one or two discussions I had during the last two weeks with a Protestant pastor who preaches from the pulpit in one of the churches in Pondicherry. He wanted to understand some of the implications of Sri Aurobindo's and Mother's philosophy, and he put to me certain questions regarding the connotation of terms which mean one thing in Christian theology and something quite different in Sri Aurobindo's philosophy.

Let us be clear regarding certain key terms that we are using. As you are aware, there is first an Absolute, a Reality, which cannot be described in words, which is infinite, which is ineffable. When the Reality reveals itself to our uplooking human intelligence, the highest human mind receives it as an eternal self-existence, which is not an inert existence but a fully conscious, self-aware Existence. It is a Consciousness, and the nature of this Consciousness is Bliss, uncaused Delight. So the Absolute Reality reveals itself to the human consciousness as Existence, Consciousness, Bliss.

Now this triune Reality as related to this universe that is its manifestation, appears in another set of three at the next level. It is the Self that sustains everything — what in Indian philosophy is called the *Atman.* It is there behind every creature, every formation, as the bedrock of that formation. This is the Self, whether on an individual basis or on a cosmic basis. Second, there is the conscious Being, the Spirit that takes cognisance, the *Purusha*, the Person. Third, there is God, the Divine Being, Ishwara.

Now this triple presentation, this self-revelation of the Reality as the Self, as the conscious Being, as God the Divine Being, has, when looked at from the point of its working, three powers, each relative to the particular manifestation. When it is the Self that bases all existence, the power that acts — the Self itself as Power — it is the conceptively creative puissance called Maya. Mark that Maya, in the pristine, original Indian tradition, does not mean a power of illusion. It means rather the power that conceives, and in the very act of conception, it formulates. It comes from the root, 'ma', to measure; it measures the immeasurable. It brings out the finite from the Infinite. This element of cleverness, of cunning, in bringing out measured formations from what is truly immeasurable has given it the name *maya.*

As from the point of the conscious being, the *Purusha*, the same power, becomes the executive power. Either what the *Purusha* wills or what it would impose on the *Purusha*, is the executive power, the *Prakriti*, that functions. Just as at the level of the Divine Being, Ishwara, God, the executive Power is *Shakti.*

So these three sets — Atman, Purusha, Ishwara; Maya, Prakriti and Shakti. He and he himself as She are not separate. Like the sun and the sunlight, the fire and the power of burning, is God and his Shakti, Purusha and his Prakriti, the Self and his Maya.

After this clarification, I was asked by the pastor why we fight shy of the term "God" and use the word "Divine". I explained to him that as far as the Mother was concerned, she preferred to avoid the word "God" in view of the traditional associations in the West with the concept of God. God has been imaged, in the West and also in some traditions in the East, in the figure of man, something anthropomorphic. He is given qualities limited by this expression; he is something like a huge man. Now Mother wanted to cut away from this association; that is why she chose to use the word "Divine".

Next the pastor asked, "What do you call 'Truth'? What is exactly the connotation of Truth?" Well, Truth is not the truth referred to in ethics or morality. Speaking the truth is not the same as the Truth in philosophy. Truth, in philosophy, at any rate in our philosophy, means the reality of things. What is Real, whether it is apparent or not, that is Truth. Ultimately, it is the Divine that is Real, therefore the Divine is the Truth and the Truth is the Divine.

Third, he asked, "What is the content of the term 'surrender' that you use?" He said that the word 'surrender' is not there in the Bible though in other Christian writings, later on, the word occurs. But the connotation is always one of defeat, of going under. I explained to him that when Sri Aurobindo used the word 'surrender' as an Indian concept, he had said "The English word 'surrender' can only inadequately render the meaning that I have in mind". What Sri Aurobindo and the Mother mean when they speak of surrender — it is not the meaning that the Oxford dictionary gives — is that it is an attitude of self-giving, self-consecration, a working out of the impulses and the determination to put oneself in tune with something else. Self-giving, self-offering, self-consecration — this is the content of surrender.

With this background, I think we can take up today the chapter from *The Synthesis*, "The Modes of the Self". You know now what the Self is. The Self that we speak of is not that vague entity spoken of in books, behind our psychological being, but the eternal Being behind the whole manifestation. It is that Self that gives meaning to everything that is built, or builds itself around it. When the disciple in one of the oldest Upanishads approaches his teacher, he asks, "Speak to me of That, by knowing which all this will be known." So that Self — the Self of all creation — That is to be known. It is to be known not in an intellectual way, not by having mental ideas, metaphysical conceptions, but seen, known and held in the consciousness. That is true knowledge; all else is mental baggage.

When, by means appropriate to this kind of knowledge, the consciousness absorbs the nature of the Self and is one with it, at some point at least to begin with, that is knowledge. Naturally the knowledge of that which is above the mind can only be got by a faculty which is above the mind. But that does not mean that one has to wait till one crosses the mind in his yoga; we all have points of contact, centres of consciousness, which are even now, at this stage open or openable to those higher planes from where this knowledge is obtained. It is possible — by silencing the mind, by lighting up the fire of aspiration in the heart — to receive the knowledge of the Self intuitively, in flashes, or as a slow revelation. A solid mass builds itself in the consciousness and one simply becomes aware of it. It is more concrete than any knowledge that one can build with the help of logic and reason.

One has to start with certain mental conceptions, true, but one can't stop there. The first step, the first part of this knowledge of the Self is to realise that not only is each form the Self in essence, but all together are part of the Self. The Self is not exhausted by any number of forms or formations; it is looming over all the forms, but on that account, the forms, the individual souls are not a bit less true than the Self. They are, in fact, projections of the Self. The individual unit, the individual soul, has an intrinsic reality which is of the same order, in essence, as that of the Self.

It was fashionable, in Indian philosophical history — and, as a matter of fact, in Asian history also — among the Buddhists, for instance, to say that there is no soul as such. They said that it was merely a bundle of sensations, *sanskaras* — at the physical level, the life level, the mental level — all held together by the thread of desire; that creates an illusion of a substantive entity. The followers of an extreme

Monism also tended, in practice — whatever they may have said in theory — to devalue the status of the soul by saying that it has no real, independent existence. It thinks it exists, it imagines it lives, but the moment knowledge dawns, like the waking up from a dream, it finds that it exists no more. It has disappeared in the Brahman.

Now these are rather extreme views which perhaps have certain justification in certain types of spiritual experience, which are certainly not the ultimate. But the point is that each soul is a projection of the Self. The Divine Reality consents to reflect itself on so many planes of existence as souls, soul existences.

Sri Aurobindo recalls the protest of a devotee, a lover of God, who insisted upon maintaining the identity by saying that he wanted to eat sugar, not become sugar. This gives in a nutshell the whole *raison d'etre* of manifestation, from a certain angle. The Divine spreads itself out, throws itself out in a thousand fragments in order that It can have the delight of union, the bliss of union with what is apparently separate from Itself. That is called the play. Someone asked the other day, "Why do they call it *Lila*, play?" That is because it is a game of the One bifurcating itself into two and more and getting together again in order to have the thrill, the joy of union. So this Reality of the individual soul against the background of the Self is a point to be remembered.

Next, this Self that is manifesting has three statuses. When projected in my soul which is active, which is participating in life, it is called the mutable purusha, the mutable Self. It changes, it participates in experience, it grows. It lends itself to all kinds of mutation as part of its experience. But the mutable purusha is not all; if it were, one would go on always mutating. Behind this mutable Self, there is the reserve of the immutable Self. There is an immense reservoir of Silence, of Power, of Bliss of which only a fraction descends and acts in the mutable. As one grows spiritually in this dynamic yoga of fulfillment, one does touch certain depths of this immutable Self where one feels free from involvements but it is not a non-existence, a full charge of power is held there in reserve. These two — the mutable self and behind it the immutable — strike the human mind as opposite poles, irreconcilable opposites. But to a higher knowledge, to a perception that goes beyond the vision of the logical reason, there is a third status, the status of the Supreme Purusha, the Transcendent, in which both meet. In fact both the mutable and the immutable are complementary aspects of the Transcendent when He turns towards the manifestation.

Each individual in this line of yoga has to realise these three possible statuses of the manifesting Self and once one realises them there is no more warring of philosophies. It is common among philosophers to argue, debate and oppose. Some say that All is One, there is only God, there is only the Divine and that is the only Truth; man is not, the world is not, so when one realises the Truth there is only the Divine and nothing else. Other philosophers say that not Monism but Dualism is the nature of the Reality; there is always a dichotomy between God and man, soul and nature, heaven and earth; whatever the state of his realisation, man cannot become one with God. This is common both to certain schools of Indian philosophy as well as to Christian thought. It is a blasphemy for them to say that man can become one with God. Here in India there are certain fanatics who would cut you down if you were to say that man can one day evolve to the status of God. They deny it. They concede that you may develop a nature which resembles His, acquire a salvation that takes you near His presence, perhaps live in the same world as He does, but becoming one with Him — you never can. Then there is a third school which is called qualified Monism, which says that it is true man is created by God; he is not a separate entity; he is dependent upon God. Both man and nature are dependent upon God, but they are always separate. This, too, has its own adherents.

Now Sri Aurobindo says that the three answers lead to three distinct possibilities of experience and realisation. One can have all these realisations in one's life. At a certain level of experience, one can feel and enjoy the relation of being separate from God — being the lover of God, the servant of God, the instrument of God. But that does not shut one out from the possibility, the reality of being — in another plane, in another poise — one with the Divine. So all the three realisations are possible for a conscious human soul to realise in the same life. In fact, for a fulfilled, fully realised being — say one who holds the Divine Consciousness, like the Mother or Sri Aurobindo, all the three realisations are simultaneously active and living.

There is another aspect of the modes of the Self and that is the personal and the impersonal. Here again, the contradictions are only posed by the limited mind. The Divine Self has all the qualities, can put out any number of qualities from itself, but all the while it is free from those qualities; the qualities do not limit it. Similarly, it can throw itself in action, but also it can remain free from action. It is because of this inherent freedom to act or not act, to manifest or not manifest a quality, that it is capable of infinite variety of action, infinite variety of quality. Similarly, whether the Supreme is a Person or an Impersonal state — say Power, Peace, Bliss — this also is a mental problem. For one who has a sufficiently comprehensive spiritual realisation, the question appears merely academic because both the personal and the impersonal are truths of the Divinity. The impersonal is a state of existence; the personal is the existent. The existence of what? Of Him who exists. So the personal is there, but the base is an impersonal state. The personal projection or formation does not exhaust the possibility; the demarcations of personality just fade away into the impersonality that is the base.

The integral seeker must start with the authentic knowledge given by those who have obtained that knowledge in life, that all these modes of experience are true and real. My experience of one mode does not preclude your experience of another mode, or preclude my own future experience of another possible mode. All these modes, the personal and the impersonal, the active and the passive, the qualitied and the unqualitied are true. Similarly the mutable, the immutable and the transcendent — all these are to be taken into account when you consider the relations of the Self with this phenomenal world which is not really a creation, but a projection, of the Supreme Self.

Any questions?

What is meant by the term Yogamaya?

The term is used in a Tantric context. *Yogamaya* in the Tantras means the power of formation that the Yogic Shakti takes. It is a way of calling *Yogashakti*, the yoga-power. Here when we use the word *Maya* instead of Shakti, it emphasises the aspect of unexpected wonders, unexpected results being turned out by the yoga-force.

Does the Supreme Self project itself into individuals?

Yes, the Supreme Self projects itself in the innumerable individual souls as also in innumerable collectivities. In the individual, the soul starts forming earlier, but in the collectivity, since the consciousness is not so much articulate, the soul takes time to form. But even the collective soul is a purposeful projection of the manifesting Soul of the universe. It is a part of it intended to bring out, to express, a certain special stress of that particular group of souls that are living in that collectivity.

Speaking of the group-soul, I was very much amused when, about three weeks ago, I received a letter from one of the institutions, newly formed I believe, in the United States. They had come to know that I had taken up the editorship of the *World Union* journal, and they wrote a nice letter, welcoming me and assuring me of their cooperation. I liked that very much, and then at the end they said, "You speak of the group-soul, which we are sure means human nature; we will have plenty to collaborate."

Certainly the group-soul is not human nature. They think: human nature is the same everywhere, so there is a certain commonalty which gives a ground for all to work together.

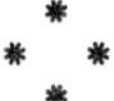

There can't be an exact correspondence between different systems. The mutable, the immutable and the transcendent are terms used in the Gita and Sri Aurobindo refers to them in the context of the Gita. But if your mind can be a little flexible I would say the psychic being, which is involved in evolution, participating in experience, acting and reacting, known or unknown to you, may be equated for the purpose of our understanding with the inner mutable purusha. But behind the psychic, there is the Self which is unmoved, which does not participate, but witnesses everything, that is the immutable. And still above there is what Sri Aurobindo would call the central being overseeing the whole affair. That perhaps could answer the description of the transcendent in the context. The psychic is in front, the Self behind, the *Jivatman*, the central being above. It is a projection of that central being which is released into the cycle of evolution that forms the soul or the psychic being.

This triple truth — mutable, immutable and transcendent — repeats itself at every level. In our mind, for instance, there is a part of the mind which is active, there is a part of the mind which is silent, there is a still deeper part which holds both together and coordinates them. So at every level, mind, life, body, there is a part which is involved, a part which supports, a part which presides over it.

The first step for all of us is to become conscious of the part which is not involved. After being conscious we must keep always a part of our consciousness or awareness in that uninvolved part and from there function so that there is a practical bifurcation in the being, — one part frontally acting, the other watching and supporting, untired, uninvolved, from behind.

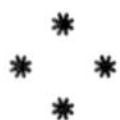

The outer vital purusha, the inner vital purusha and the Divine Being presiding over the vital manifestation.

We will be coming, I think, in one of the later chapters to know how the Divine Self is manifest in all the three statuses at each level. So it is the one Self that is called at different levels, the mental purusha, the vital purusha, the physical purusha and on each level, again, the outer being, the inner being and the deepest.

Is it possible to become aware of the transcendent?

As long as our awareness is confined to the surface, it is not possible. But in our own being there is a level which is transcendent of this manifestation. Each one of us has a station in the transcendent but we are not conscious of it. Once, however, we develop an integral, multiple consciousness and become aware of all the dimensions that are possible for the manifest consciousness, that transcendent status lends itself to be felt and experienced. It is not that you can't experience it; it is not involved, not affected, in the movement of manifestation, the movement of the universe, but it supports it. It is not aloof; it is not turned away, it supports.

That is the difference between Shankara's philosophy and Sri Aurobindo's. Sri Aurobindo says that the Absolute is not turned away from the Universe. The universe has been projected from the Absolute and the Absolute supports it and it is possible, if only one develops a multiple consciousness, to become aware of this. It comprehends both horizontally and vertically the full extent of the Being and the Becoming.

Should we not do our best to build up world unity?

The world-mind is rapidly turning towards this realisation of unity. We do not have to build this world unity by human effort. The Mother says that the world unity has been fashioned already; it is ready at the doors of the physical universe, waiting for the veil to be removed. The veil consists of the human egoism, and the refusal on the part of each nation to give up its attitude of division. That is why nature is forcing nations to come together, whether in clash or in harmony, it does not matter. They are being brought together, shocked into oneness.

It was inconceivable, say twenty years ago, that this much of oneness, unity could be possible. If today sworn enemies like America and China can sit together at the table to discuss matters, if Russia and America leaving aside points of dispute, can meet in the areas of agreement, that surely is a pointer. I do not agree with people who say that the U.N.O. is a failure and it has to be abolished. Sri Aurobindo warned us against this facile assumption long ago. He said that the League of Nations was doomed to go because of its inherent contradictions, so another cataclysm became inevitable and the U.N.O. came. If the U.N.O. has to go and another world-body take its place, it means another world war has to come. But with the descent of the Truth-Consciousness in 1956, a world conflagration can safely be ruled out. There may be local battles and wars of which one realises the futility on the third or the fourth day and the forces of harmony again bring them together. But there cannot be a world war; there is no alternative to the U.N.O. The U.N.O. has to be mended and not ended, and there is an acceptance of this approach at the top levels, whether in the Communist block or the non-Communist block.

There is no alternative. And if the yogic transformation that is being precipitated in the Mother's body goes at its expected speed, it is bound to have repercussions even at the political level of human unity. Almost the very phrases and expressions which we use here, we read in journals that are being published in the States. Well, how do you explain that? There is already an impact in the realm of ideas. They may say we are borrowing their expressions; we may say they are borrowing ours, but the truth is that the Truth is descending and whoever is open becomes aware of certain expressions, because they are the *mots justes*, the right words for the truths that are descending.

This yoga is a collective yoga and not an individual yoga. So even our minus contributions affect humanity adversely. Here is a kind of focus where anything that happens has its reactions on a larger scale. Greater harmony and understanding between inmates, whether in the Ashram or in Auroville, will be a positive factor towards the change of consciousness in humanity. Growth of falsehood, disharmony and ill-will, and a lack of faith amongst us will delay the consummation on the universal scale. Our behaviour would not at all matter for the collective evolution of the world if we were living elsewhere. It is because here a concentrated force is operating that all of us, who constitute the field of that force, take on a certain representative character, and we have a certain responsibility to our Maker, who has brought us here, who is maintaining us here, to keep up our part of the implied agreement.

9

The Realisation of Saccidananda

All of you, doubtless, read and, I hope, pondered over the message given by Mother for the special day yesterday. Each word represents a concept. There is first:

Beyond man's consciousness,

The whole message is an invocation. You will ask, invocation of what? It is a call to the Supreme Reality, and that Reality cannot be attained by the human consciousness as it is. The mind of man, as it is today, cannot reach it. As graphically described in one of the ancient Upanishads, the mind falls back. It tries to reach it, but it just falls back. It cannot soar on its own wings; it returns baffled. Supposing, by some supreme effort, the sanction of Grace, the human consciousness — not the mind — can reach out to it, find a link with it, enter into communion with it and realise it in a way; it will still be unable to express it; it is ineffable. Here, again, another seer of the Upanishad has described how speech falls dumb when it is face to face with that Reality. It is inaccessible to the human mind, ineffable to the human speech. Next comes:

O, Thee

Because it is inaccessible, because it is ineffable, it is not an abstraction. It is not some philosopher's Absolute of the conceptual frame. It is not simply That; it is also Thee. It is a Supreme Consciousness — alive, embodied, capable of having relations, capable of responding. That is why she calls it "Thee". It is a dynamic, individualised Presence which lends itself in its own way. It is an embodied Consciousness in a supreme integrality, higher than the highest in this creation.

Unique Reality,

It is a Reality that is sole; one without a second. For there cannot be another. There is one indestructible Reality which pervades everything, which contains everything. All that you see and do not see is this Reality in principle and in manifestation.

Divine Truth.

The nature of this Reality is Truth; that bedrock of Truth which constitutes the stuff of all existence, governs all movement. It is what *is*.

In this short invocation, all the viewpoints of philosophers, of seers, have been integrated. It is not merely impersonal, but also personal. Not a negative Absolute, not a negative Transcendent, but a positive, Divine, Unique Truth that constitutes all existence.

This gives a very fine background to our theme today — "The realisation of Saccidananda". *Sat* is Existence; *Chit* is Consciousness; *Ananda* is Delight of Existence. We have considered, last time, the various modes of the Self — the personal and the impersonal, the qualitied and the unqualitied, the One and the Many. We have discussed threadbare the different poises, statuses taken by the Reality when it is turned to manifestation. When it is in itself, concentrated in itself, it is impossible for us to know what it is. That is why it is simply described as "That". But when it is turned towards the manifestation, it reveals itself in a triple poise; Existence that is Consciousness; Consciousness whose nature is Delight.

Everything in the universe, of which we are a part, resolves itself, ultimately, into an existence. Even when a particular form is dissolved, it does not disappear; it disappears from that particular form, but the stuff remains. Each part goes back to its matrix. If a human form, for instance, is dissolved, the physical body is reabsorbed into the universal Matter, the life-energy rejoins the ocean of the flow of Life-Force, the Mind is sucked back into the Universal

Mind, and the soul temporarily withdraws itself into the psychic world. Nothing is lost. The perception of the ancients that nothing is destroyed, everything is indestructible, has been amply confirmed by the discoveries of modern science of the indestructibility of matter and energy. All that has been perceived and conceived from one end is being slowly and gradually confirmed from the other end.

Now this Existence pervades all that is manifest and, where things are not manifest, what is called unmanifest, it is something that is unmanifest. There is an existence; there *is*. If man has the temerity to deny, if he says there is no existence, he becomes as one described in one of the ancient Upanishads in a terrible idiom, "He who thinks It is not, himself becomes the Not". He covers himself with negation, he cancels himself from the flow of life, from manifestation, and he is withdrawn. But he who affirms It is, he affirms himself in that Reality.

This Existence, *Sat*, is not a monotone. It holds in its bosom the whole of infinity. It is its self-extension in what we call space that is called infinity, self-extension in duration that is called eternity. Whether it is time or space they are but terms of something that exists, something projects itself.

And the nature of this Existence is a Supreme Consciousness, called in the Indian philosophy *Chit*. Consciousness, — not simply something that is aware and nothing more, but a dynamic awareness. It is a Consciousness that is at the same time a Force. What it conceives it can execute; what it perceives it can work out. At a certain level this knowledge and will, vision and actualisation, are simultaneous. This Consciousness — the Divine Consciousness in manifestation — formulates itself on different levels in suitable forms, forms that are apposite and suitable to the organisation of things on each level.

Thus, for instance, we have the mind. Now certainly nobody would say that our mind constitutes the entire range of consciousness in us. Whatever some psychologists may say, mind is a very small and tiny fragment of the consciousness that is extended in us. Mind is a particular formation. As it functions today, it is ideative, conceptual, organising and coordinating the sensations, but that formulation is only on the surface. Behind, there is the larger formulation of consciousness which we call the subliminal; below there is what we call the subconscious — a level where consciousness is mostly absorbed and is only half-awake in the human sense. Below the sub-consciousness are belts of the unconscious, where things are differently held. It is not that consciousness is not there; consciousness is there — consciousness does function, but at a rate of vibration, in a way of functioning that cannot be caught by our awareness. It is below our seizing apparatus. But on that account we cannot say that there is no consciousness there. Below the unconscious there are regions where is a hard inconscience, nescience. Even there consciousness is but it is so much self-absorbed, so much lost in itself, that it looks as if it were not there. But there is no element, not an atom on earth, where consciousness is not.

As in the individual, so in the universe, consciousness is spread out in various gradations. Below the mental level of man there is the animal level; consciousness is organised in a different way. Below the animal level, there is the plant level and the vegetable level. Below that is the metal and stone; everywhere there is consciousness. Two thousand years ago it was Manu, the legendary thinker, the first man, who said, "All these are awake within; there is a consciousness in all."

As at the level of man and below, there are gradations and gradations of consciousness, so above, in the upper hemisphere of existence; consciousness is severally organised and manifest. Beyond the highest heights of the mind is what Sri Aurobindo calls the Supermind, the supramental consciousness, where the whole of consciousness is so formulated that the One and the Many are simultaneously active. The One is always aware that it is the soul of the Many; the Many are always aware that they are based on the One. There is an automatic execution of what one thinks — no, there is no thinking there, — of what one sees, what one knows, Knowledge-Will, Real-Idea — these are different expressive names given to this organisation of consciousness at the Truth level by Sri Aurobindo. Beyond are the domains of sheer Consciousness, only *Chit.*

There is no question there of creation; everything is aware, supremely aware of what is, what is to happen. It is a throb of Consciousness. When analysed, this Consciousness — and it lends itself to be scrutinised on the higher levels more easily than on the lower ones — is seen to be of the nature of Bliss. Where the Consciousness is active in its own right without having to be interpreted by the human mind, there there is a spontaneous vibration of Bliss because the nature of Existence is Bliss. Wherever there is Existence, there is Ananda.

If today in our little world of earth we find so much of pain, so much of suffering, it is because in our situation, caused by division in our consciousness, by limitation of our life-force, we have isolated ourselves from the ocean of Life-Force, from the waves of Ananda that beat above. Anything beyond what we can grasp and bear impinges upon us as pain. If, by some means, we develop the capacity of enlargement, of extending our area of consciousness, the same impingements will evoke different vibrations from us. Even as it is — Sri Aurobindo points out in his *Life Divine* — the sum total of happiness in the world is much more than the sum total of pain; otherwise, man simply could not exist.

After all is said and done, nobody wants to die. Even people who say they want to die are always preparing to escape death. That is because the claim of the delight within to assert itself, to enjoy the field given to it by the Divine is asserted. It is a crime against the Maker, a crime against oneself to think of ending one's life. It is not a question of sin or merit; the soul has chosen life and if, due to some disappointment, failure, frustration, we think of ending our life, it is an offence to the divine element within us which has come to express the Delight. If we fail, because of our limitations and ignorance, it is our failure, not the failure of God.

Whom are you going to punish? Always the motive behind suicide is to punish — punish someone who loves you, punish someone whom you feel has been unfair to you, punish even God, whom you feel to be the author of your misery. But as the Mother points out, immediately after leaving the body you begin to struggle. It is an unnatural exit; you try to get back, but there is no physical body to protect you. All kinds of malevolent and evil forces and beings rush upon you to seize you and eat you up. You try to rush back to the protection of the physical body, but you don't have it. The divine protection is ineffective, because you have negated and denied it. So, after you go through this post-mortem misery and are somehow dragged into the place of rest, in the next incarnation you are obliged to start at that precise moment where you forcibly interrupted the soul's experience. And invariably the circumstances into which you are born in the next birth are worse — they call for more suffering and impose upon you a harder test than was given in the previous birth.

All this is a side issue, but the fact remains that pain is unnatural, suffering is unnatural, that is why we feel it all the more. When one is just happy, one doesn't even know that one is happy; one just takes it for granted. And that is right; it is natural. The unnatural condition of pain is caused by our self-limitation. We hide ourselves behind the walls of our ego wanting to guard our so-called independence, wanting to function separately from others, and when the whole universal life floods upon us, we react in pain. When it is physical it is pain; when it is mental it is suffering. Either way, it is an unnatural condition caused by one's self-limitation and remediable by the enlargement of consciousness, by delving within oneself and finding the stream of uncaused bliss flowing at the level of the soul. The psychic region is the gate through which to enter into this domain of bliss.

These then — *Sat, Chit, Ananda* — are the basic terms of this manifestation. On every level, at every gradation, all these are there. That is how what is called the *siddhi* of delight can be realised at the physical level, at the vital level, at the mental level. You must have heard — I do not know how many have seen — that there are in India ascetics who are not at all mentally developed. You will find some on the roadside, on dung heaps where they live in a different consciousness. They have no high spiritual culture, they will not understand that language, but still they have what is called a *siddhi*, fulfillment on the physical plane.

Now how is it possible, you may ask, for a man to realise that *Ananda* stage if he does not proceed from level to level? Well, when you choose this Integral Yoga on the line of spiritual evolution, that is the procedure. But if you are satisfied in realising God, in realising God's power and bliss on the physical plane, that is quite possible. By Hathayoga, by concentrating on the physical body, by galvanising all the physical energies, by mobilising the stream of physical consciousness and evoking the Divine Self that is situate on the physical plane, it is possible to realise the Divine Consciousness in the physical. The mind, the vital and all other planes are dead to such a yogi. He does not care for spiritual evolution; his soul has not come for it. He seeks his way of escape, his way of withdrawal, from the cycle of manifestation at the physical level and he gets it and is satisfied.

Similarly, there are saints who have realised the Divine on the emotional level. They are devotees, minstrels of God, who sing the praise of God, who can thrill you into an awareness of the Delight of God. They ignore the physical, they do not care for knowledge, for philosophy — they say it is all dry. All that they concentrate upon is feeling the Divine Presence within themselves. Some extend that awareness to feel the Divine around them — in man, in the animal, in the trees, in the stone pillars, everywhere. They see the one Cosmic Divine and the whole body, the whole being, is inundated with vibrations of delight at the fact that the Divine is manifest. They realise the Divine Consciousness, the consciousness of the Divine Delight, in their heart. Outwardly, they have absolutely no control.

You call them "freaks". They do not answer to the intention of the creator. They do not follow the noble line of ascent to God that has been forged by the Divine in man. They are aberrations choosing either to cancel themselves into Nirvana or to withdraw at certain levels of their evolution as they choose.

There are many kinds of movements raging, at the moment, in the West. Somewhere they have a true basis, but as they are being propagated, as they are being practised, it is nothing but a vital play. Everyone gets a vital thrill; they just feel wild with the influx and the infusion of the vital energies, not all of which are healthy. They feel they are in contact with the Divine; actually they have only opened themselves to the vital world. Possibly among a thousand who follow, it may be one or two who may have got linked with the Divine manifest at the emotional centre.

So whichever plane you exist upon, whichever is the dominating truth for you, there you can realise the Divine. That is because this triple principle of *Saccidananda* is embedded at every level of creation.

Speaking of saints, devotion, I am tempted to narrate to you two stories — which are not quite stories for I have reason to believe they have some basis in fact. I was reading a particular book on the great saint Ramanuja who founded the system of qualified Monism just as Shankara founded the system of Monism, *advaita.* Ramanuja came to controvert it, and he asserted the reality of the universe, the reality of life, the reality of manifestation. He said, man and God are separate entities, but man is dependent upon God. Now for the first story: Once when Ramanuja was travelling on foot — he had not yet become the supreme pontiff — he heard that a particular devotee who was attending to a deity in the temple was so intimate with the God of that temple that he could converse with him. So he went to his house and asked him, "I hear that you talk to Lord Srinivasa at night". The devotee said, "Yes". "Then do you mind asking him if I will get self-realisation in this birth?" asked Ramanuja. The devotee said, "Certainly I shall ask; come tomorrow morning, I will give you his reply."

Now this devotee was a singer. He used to compose and sing many songs and once, when pleased with him, Lord Srinivasa had asked him, "What boon shall I give you?" and he had said, "When I sing, you should dance." The deity agreed. And thereafter the devotee would close the doors of the temple and sing and that image would come alive and dance.

That night after Ramanuja had left, the devotee went into the temple and asked his god whether Ramanuja would get realisation. Lord Srinivasa replied, "Yes, tell him that I have brought him into birth this time precisely to give him self-realisation." Then the devotee said, "What about me, when will I get self-realisation?" Lord Srinivasa said, "why self-realisation for you? How does the question arise?" The devotee answered, "Well, I am singing to you, I am doing it daily." "You sing and I dance; that is what you wanted." was the Lord's reply.

This is what the Mother calls bargaining. Once we determine the way in which the response has to come, the responsibility of the Divine ceases. We get what we want, but we shut ourselves from the Grace. When we give, it should be unconditional; devotion, love, service, should be absolutely unconditional.

Now another story of the same saint. When he settled down in the South, as a pontiff, he had many disciples, one of whom was specially devoted to him. That man would spend all the twenty-four hours with the saint; he would not go home. Naturally his mother and wife were very troubled. So the mother went to the guru and said to him, "Sir we have absolutely no objection to our son serving you, but you must know that he is in a householder's position. He has got a wife, a family to look after and the family deities to worship. What is going to happen? We have no children at home and according to the *shastras* unless there is a child in the family, the family fortunes are affected. So you must send him home at least at night; in the morning you can have him back." Ramanuja thought that the mother's complaint was just. So he called his disciple and said, "Look here, what your mother says is perfectly true. You are still in the status of a householder, and the responsibility of a householder binds you. I can't stand between that and you. You must go back and fulfill your householder's duties; then I will give you *sannyasa*, (vows of renunciation) — not before that. The disciple replied, "You are the teacher, I will do what you say; I have no other alternative, but please listen to my difficulty. Ever since I have come and started serving you, something has been growing in my heart. There is a light that is gradually spreading. The figure of the Lord, as it is in the image in the temple, is becoming clearer day by day. So at every moment when I am not busy or talking to people, I see that brilliant, luminous face looking at me, smiling at me; not for a moment when I am alone am I without it. So when he is regarding me like that all the time, how can you expect me to do an animal act in his presence? I can't think of indulging myself in his divine Presence." The teacher was struck; he said, "Yes, you are right". He called for those ladies and explained to them that his disciple had gone beyond the normal human level, and he told them, "I have to relieve him of the responsibilities of the householder." The very next day Ramanuja gave him *sannyasa*, made him an ascetic and freed him from his normal responsibilities.

This is not merely a story; it is based on real spiritual experience. It is impossible for a man to imagine these things. There are states of consciousness when you feel very close to Mother, when you feel that Mother is in every part of your body; at that moment — or when you think of those conditions — it is just impossible for you to indulge in any lower movement, either of greed, sex or any other kind of dissipation.

The story emphasises that one has to concentrate on the positives, on bringing down the glories of God, activising the purity, the light, the knowledge. All the opposites just drop away. Instead of struggling with the dark entities, trying to clear the decks, one has to concentrate upon the positive side. The negative just drops off.

Questions and Answers

Question: *Is sex to be considered an animal act?*

Answer: It depends how you regard it. That particular person felt that sex was an animal function. If one has developed a consciousness where every human activity — including sex — assumes its rightful aspect of an outflowing of the divine Energy, the Divine Consciousness, then certainly sex is not an animal act.

This was the ideal that had been placed before the seekers in the Tantras, before it was usurped by the cunning vital which turned it into indulgence of sex under the label of spirituality. It all depends upon one's sincerity. If one has developed that purity, by which sex becomes a process of communicating, of receiving the pure bliss of the delight of existence, there is nothing to be said against it. But this entails an extraordinary amount of purity. The body cannot vibrate in the gross sense.

What Sri Aurobindo describes in one of his letters as the vibrations of chaos, the vibrations of loss of control over oneself — it is these that are unspiritual. If those vibrations can be kept out, if sex can be experienced in the poise of peace, with absolute detachment, purely as a channel and a communication of the feeling of oneness, a feeling of self-giving, then certainly, like every other activity of life, sex is not an animal operation. But the sex books describe and people speak about sex as it is indulged in normally at the human level. It is another matter whether one who has arrived at a superhuman level cares for sex. I have known very highly developed seekers, sadhaks, who — they were householders — after going through the ritual of sex as prescribed for a God-seeking householder in the Tantras, found that by the time they arranged all those rituals, recited the mantras and invocations, the normal sex was just not there. So sex is all right for Rishis and other realised men who do it for the sake of procreation. But sex as sex, sex as something that gives that thrill of enjoyment in the physical plane, does not exist at that level. It becomes a nuisance.

Ultimately, it depends upon one's sincerity whether sex is animal or divine.

10

The Difficulties of the Mental Being

Normally I inform Mother in the morning the day we are to meet here. But for the past few weeks she is, as you all know, in a state of consciousness that discourages us from talking to her. So before I entered her room, I said to her in my mind that that evening I was to go to Auroville, but I didn't express it verbally to her. But as she was picking up flowers for me, she picked up the flower "Auroville" and said, 'Hmm'. It moved me very much; and there we are.

The subject for our discussion this evening is "The Difficulties of the Mental Being". We have traversed a considerable portion of the Yoga of Knowledge; we have seen that the object is first to detach oneself from involvement in the life of the senses, withdraw from the sense mind and poise after poise, to arrive at the status of the pure self. That is the first step. We have also seen that after arriving at the pure Self, one has to ascend the ladder of the being and seek to realise the Supreme Self, or Brahman, as they call it in the ancient Indian tradition, which presents itself to the up-looking human intelligence as Saccidananda.

We have also seen that it is not enough even to realise the Supreme Existence, but it is necessary to embrace all life, the whole of the universe, in the consciousness thus attained. In other words, we seek to perceive all life through the eye of the Saccidananda.

There are certain difficulties for the human mind, constituted as it is. The human mind, the reasoning intelligence, surveys and understands in segments. When it is forced to recognise and realise the impersonal aspect of the Divine, of the Saccidananda, it shuts itself to the possibility of the Existent; it believes only in the Existence. The human mind is to be taught by the method of the Integral Yoga to arrive at a Transcendent which embraces both the personal and the impersonal, to use one as the base of the other, to use the other as the expression of the one. The personal and the impersonal, the qualitied and the non-qualitied — these are the differences and distinctions usually made by the rational intelligence which, however, do not hold good once one arrives at the level of the spiritual mind.

The mind may also be captured by the presentation of the Consciousness-Force aspect of the Supreme. It sees the tremendous charge of consciousness as force and it has the conception of the whole world as a movement of consciousness, as a projection of the force of consciousness. It is the philosophy of the Tantras, which conceives the world as a mobile expression of a self-existent consciousness. Or the mind may experience something of the Bliss, and it tends to regard the absolute Reality as the Highest state of Bliss, or Nirvana, of which the Buddha spoke. But left to itself, the mind is unable to conceive that the Reality is one in three aspects; that all the three triply constitute the Absolute.

It is due to the gulf between the mind as it is and the supreme height at which the Saccidananda is realised that this difficulty is aggravated. Sri Aurobindo points out that there are levels of consciousness in oneself above the rational intelligence which have correspondents and links with the cosmic plane which leads to Saccidananda. And if we activate those levels of consciousness within ourselves, they open our being to influences from those planes of existence — the intuitive, the illuminative, and so on — till a new consciousness is gradually built up which can absorb the Supreme Being, without deformation, without dilution.

This is as far as the ascent is concerned, but even when

the ascent is ultimately reached you are faced with a problem. You arrive at the summit — may be with the totality of the being — but the world around, the universe around remains the same. If you were to come down to function in the world you would have to leave all those states of consciousness upon their various levels and function here again on the usual material level. For that purpose there is the evocation, the calling down of the Being and the influence of Saccidananda in the human consciousness. As these states of consciousness first emanate their influences, send their messengers in appropriate form and as the human being opens himself, keeps himself receptive, allows himself to be moulded, these influences from higher up organise themselves, support the ascending movement and build up in man a totally new consciousness — the consciousness of the Knowledge-Will that is the principle of the Supramental world; the flow of causeless Bliss that is the principle of the world of Ananda; a self-existent and a dynamic Consciousness which is the principle of the Chit-world; and a sheer Existence which is eternal, which is absolute.

These are the possibilities open to the human mind, but it has to first mentally accept this organisation of the universal principles in the macrocosm as well as in the microcosm, make itself subtle and plastic, adjust itself to the revelations of the higher planes of existence as they come by the process of yoga. The difficulties are there, but if the mind gives up its rigidities, its preferences as dictated by the habit of logical reasoning, which is valid only for a small fragment of life, these difficulties can be overcome.

I knew that discussion of this subject would take only a short time, and I thought that you would be interested in hearing of a mantra given by Sri Aurobindo long, long ago — must be about forty years — to Champaklal. The latter was kind enough to show it to me, and I felt like sharing it with you all now. This is the mantra for the seeker of the Integral Path.

In the night as in the day, be always with me.
In sleep as in waking let me feel in me always
the reality of your presence.
Let it sustain and make to grow in me Truth,
Consciousness and Bliss constantly
and at all times.

Due to my Sanskritic background, whenever I see such aphoristic messages, my mind rushes to explain — first to myself, and then to others. And here is what I have written about the mantra; I hope it will be acceptable to all of you.

The Divine is invoked to be present. When? Not at this time or that, not only at periods of prayer or stress, but *always*, during all the twenty-four hours. "with me" — intimately and actively, the presence must surround and abide.

In the night as in the day be always with me.

It is not enough that the Presence is there; one must feel it and live in it. Whether one is awake and active or one is asleep and inactive, one must live in that Presence. It is only by living in that Presence during one's waking hours that the Presence can be prolonged even when one is not awake. The participation in the Presence is to be built up during the day so that it continues during the night.

It is not enough to be conscious of the Divine Presence during states of enlightenment, of soul-lit awareness, the Day. It is equally necessary to feel the Presence even during conditions of obscurity, of the darkness of tamas or temporary failure of aspiration, the Night. In both the states of the being the reality of the Divine Presence must be direct and incessant in experience.

In sleep as in waking let me feel in me always the reality of your Presence.

And what is the result of this constant Presence of the Divine in oneself? It *sustains* his aspiration, supports his effort to grow in identity with the Divine. He grows; and along with him, aiding him to grow, there forms in him the Divine

Truth. The Divine Consciousness builds itself, and with it the Divine Bliss, in his growing being. The more he enlarges himself, the deeper he awakes, the greater is the occupation of the Divine Presence in its triple way of Truth-Existence, Consciousness and Bliss. The process is constant, unbroken, whether one is fully aware of it on the surface levels of being or not.

Let it sustain and make to grow in me Truth, Consciousness and Bliss constantly and at all times.

The Divine Presence is invoked in its integrality as well as in its eternity.

From Questions and Answers

True, the Mother told someone that a new phase in her work has begun. What exactly it means each one can speculate for himself. And when she was asked further she said that nobody would understand. So I was reminded of Sri Aurobindo's line in *Savitri*: "Eternity speaks, none understands its word."

Last Sunday I had to give a talk on pretty much the same subject under the auspices of the *World Union*. I was supposed to explain the relevance of the supplement that was distributed along with the Bulletin, "The Truth to be Realised Now" — as to what it means, what is its significance. There I mentioned that it was just two or three days earlier before the talk that someone who is sensitive to these vibrations found, as she entered the Ashram building in the morning, a powerful spell of something new. She went ahead and sat for meditation. During meditation, there was a pull from above. She looked up and she saw all the gods waiting above the Ashram with all kinds of musical instruments — tamborines, cymbals, drums etc. — waiting to strike, and all looking expectantly at the Ashram in absolute silence; they were waiting. That shows what is going on behind the veil, something great is due.

I went on further to say that the gods were waiting but whether we men are waiting is another matter. So we are on the eve of something great. That's all that I can say, but whether her remark meant all this I do not know . . .

Actually Sri Aurobindo is working — not doing *some* of the work but participating in all the work that she does on earth. On his own on the subtle-physical plane, he is preparing for the whole manifestation to be organised so that at the right moment it can be precipitated on the earth. So he is there — as the Mother once explained — readying all that is to be manifested. Even those who have been working with him during so many incarnations, who were here, who have died, all are there with him, some actively participating, some silently observing, but all grouped around him. And he is actively working — more actively than when he was on earth, that's how Mother explained it.

Particularly, he is guiding the destiny of India, because it is essential for the future of humanity that the soul of India is intact and India takes the right direction, recovers her spiritual heritage. So in spite of all the bunglings and the detours taken by the leadership in various spheres of life, the Mother feels that because he is at the helm there, the ship of the State of India will arrive safe at the Port.

And what is happening is that the advanced minds of humanity have accepted the necessity of a change of consciousness, and admit the immanence of a new grade of consciousness on earth. They may give different names to it, they may lack the courage to work out what they envision, but still, the advanced minds have moved forward during the last one decade and accepted; whether they will have the courage to translate it into practice is another matter.

We know what the difficulties are. All of us have sincerely accepted the ideal of transformation of a new consciousness but we know how hard it is, the moment we start translating it into practice. If at each moment of our life we want to be true to this aspiration, we must realise what it means, where we fight shy of it, where we hide things from ourselves, where we procrastinate. If we are objective in our self-scrutiny, we know. When we in the Ashram and Auroville are what we are, we can hardly expect people in the world to wake up to their responsibility. It is for that reason that Mother expects a greater awakening on the part of those who are in this focus of the cosmic energies, cosmic forces and turn a new leaf; a step which is bound to have its consequences on a wider scale in the world.

A very real difficulty in reaching this transition between the mental consciousness and the new consciousness came up in something that I had to face which is common to all Americans here. And that is on the issuance of a new passport – not a renewal but a new passport – it is required that one swears allegiance to the constitution of the United States and to bear arms against any enemy determined by that government. And it came very forcibly to my memory that the U. S. fleet was heading towards the Bay of Bengal, and the possibility of having to bear arms against what I feel is my spiritual Motherland, India, was in the realm of possibility.

There are levels of living. The surface being lives on a practical physical-vital level, and the consciousness lives on another level which is natural to it. So in these matters where one is faced with the system, one has to balance, accept for the time being, the lesser evil. Otherwise, one has to spend all the lifetime in fighting the system.

We know that the system will change only when the consciousness at the top will change. So one has to concentrate there inwardly, and if the inner aspiration is strong, whatever the outer forms and rules, things always happen by which you will not be obliged to act in a way that is contrary to your aspiration.

When in 1939 the second world war broke out, Pavitra who was a Frenchman and an officer in the French Army was called as soon as the war started. He was summoned to come back and join his ranks. He naturally objected to war because it is contrary to this yoga, and he did not like to leave the Ashram, for Mother used to rely on him for many things. At the office in Paris, things were postponed, but ultimately the final communication came for him to don his uniform and leave immediately. Even a notice had been put up saying that new arrangements had to be made in the department as Pavitra had to leave. Mother, however, did not give up the matter. She exerted her will in her own way and at the last moment when Pavitra had to leave, the orders were withdrawn!

We have seen this in the lives of many seekers. When the law required them to do certain things which were against the preference of their soul, if they were sincere in their aspiration, something would happen by which they would be relieved of those awkward situations.

These forms and rules don't mean much in terms of spiritual consciousness. But living as we do in this world of ignorance, till the world changes its character, at certain levels we have to accept certain balancings. It does not mean that one is untrue to oneself.

11

The Passive and the Active Brahman

We spoke of the difficulties of the mental being, the difficulty that the mind has in seizing the Supreme Reality as it presents itself to the human consciousness. The difficulties are, indeed, many and the ancients have devised a number of methods to alleviate them.

To take one instance, let us start with a story, a famous story, from one of the Upanishads. There was a great sage, Varuna by name, who knew the Reality in his own way. And because he knew, there were always disciples flocking around him to learn from him what there is to be known. One morning, his own son approached him and said, "Lord, teach me of the Eternal." In those days teachers did not have books; they did not make the disciples write; they did not even verbally teach what they knew. Their method was different; it was one which we are on the verge of re-discovering today in the field of education. They believed in igniting the flame, in communicating the spark that would grow in the being of the seeker, in the being of the student.

So he called his son and said, "You wish to know the Eternal. Know that from which all things are born and being born by which they live and at the end of their living into which they pass." The boy said he would try and he concentrated his mind, brooded over the words of his father and tried to know what that is from which all things are born, by which all live, and into which all things enter upon their passing. He came back to his father after some days and said: "Food is the Eternal, for by food, it appears, all things are born, obviously by food they are sustained and into the great Food they pass." The father heard him and said, "Know the Eternal, do askesis. For askesis is the Eternal". The boy went back. Again he brooded over the Eternal in his mind, in his consciousness, and when he next went to his father, he told him, "*prana*, the life-force, is the Eternal. For from the life-force indeed are all things born, by the energy of the life-force all things are sustained, and into the great sea of life-force all beings pass." The father again said, "Do askesis, for askesis is the Eternal." The boy went back, brooded further in his consciousness and returned to his father and said, "The mind is the Eternal, for by mind, it appears, all are born, all are projected into existence, and by the mind they are maintained, and into mind they pass." Still the father said, "Do askesis, for askesis is the Eternal." Bewildered, the young seeker went back, continued his askesis, brooded further, came back and told his father, "Knowledge is the Eternal, for out of knowledge, it appears, things come into being, by knowledge they are maintained, and into knowledge they pass." "Do askesis, for askesis is the Eternal," repeated the father. And once again the boy went back, brooded over the Eternal, and when he came back next, his face was beaming with joy. He said, "Bliss is the Eternal, for out of Bliss all creation comes to be, by the underlying bliss all is sustained, and into the undying bliss all enters."

The father did not impose further askesis on the seeker, for he had, indeed, traversed the whole range of the becoming of the Eternal. The Supreme Reality manifests itself as food, as matter; as life-force, as prana; as mind, as knowledge, what we would call in our parlance Truth-Knowledge; as Bliss, what we call Ananda, about which the Upanishad says, who indeed could live if there were not this underlying Bliss sustaining the creation? But for this Bliss in the ether man could not breathe; Bliss is the essential characteristic of this creation.

If we creatures do not perceive this inalienable feature of bliss, but are constantly seized with the impacts of pain and suffering, it is because we are half-blind. We are unseeing — we have the eyes to see, but we refuse to see. We limit ourselves within the walls of our ego, guard ourselves from the impacts of the world, and when the mighty impacts from the universal forces impinge upon us, in our petty limitations we shrink. And that shrinking, translated in sensational terms, is what is called pain. If only we could enlarge ourselves, break through the walls of ignorance and ego, then every contact would be a vibration of Bliss. Sri Aurobindo refers to this legend of the realisation of Brahman, by the son of Varuna, as a capital way for the human mind to realise the Reality on each plane of being, comprehend it on each grade of consciousness.

A seeker must integrate himself in the lower grade before he goes into the next, and then cover, step by step, plane by plane, the graded becomings of the Brahman, till he arrives at the highest. By so doing he leaves out nothing. He realises the Divine Existence, the Divine Soul in itself, also the divine becoming, the Nature-Soul. So in both the aspects, the passive and the active, he realises the Divine Reality.

There are, indeed, other ways of realising the Supreme. We have seen how, in the yoga of knowledge, the aspirant withdraws his gaze from the outer objects, detaches his consciousness from the objects of ego and desire after which the senses and the mind run. Then after a certain degree of detachment is arrived at, he turns his gaze inward, locates the centre of his Self, and becomes aware of his inner being.

In the first stages, when one thus becomes aware of the Self as detached from nature, from the million formulations of nature, the poise in which the Self reveals itself is one of witness. It observes, it watches, but it does not involve itself. As one's identification with the witness Self deepens, the poise changes, the Self puts on an aspect of greater immobility, a silence in which nothing moves. It does not even look at what is going on, it is self-absorbed, silent, austere, alone. When one stations oneself in the bosom of that Silence, that Self, all seem figures, figments, names and forms moving about, — and they all look lifeless.

As one pursues one's quest still deeper, one comes to an area where everything is unknown and unknowable. The mental faculties just drop; only the consciousness is awake, and the mind realises that it cannot know. When it looks at the world from that station, all looks unreal. All looks like froth on the surface of the ocean. It is possible to realise the Reality in this aspect but one must remember it is only an aspect.

Further, this unknown and the unknowable can be realised, according to the bent of the soul, either as an Absolute Reality, sheer Existence, or as a Non-Existence, a nihil, a zero in which everything disappears.

These are certain types of realisation that you can have in the quest for the Reality. Whichever way you pursue the quest in this line, the world is left out, the universe remains what it is, you are absorbed in your Self. This way, certainly, is not open to the seeker of the Integral Truth.

It is possible for the seeker, after he has detached himself from the outer preoccupations, to ascend to the heights of his own spiritual mind, realise the pure Existence there, on the heights of the mind, and project himself in the universe in the way of the becoming of the Self, and realise the same Self as the All — all is an expression of that Self. Not merely that, he sees that each form has a certain reality because the Self informs each form. In each, there is the indwelling Self. The Self is in each, the Self is there as each — it fills the universe. And it is not yet exhausted; it transcends.

It is possible, in knowledge, to grasp this Reality. But in practice, in day to day life, one is apt to lose oneself in the mechanics of Nature. One loses oneself in Nature only as long as one looks upon Nature as something foreign to the Self. In the philosophy of the Sankhya the whole creation is regarded in terms of Soul and Nature. There is one mighty Nature which is self-operative, self-existent, mechanical in its movements, but there are a million souls and the activity of Nature is reflected in the individual Self that watches. The very watching, the very witnessing of the Soul operates as a sanction for Nature. And their philosophy is that once you awake to this state of things and detach yourself, refuse the sanction of the Soul, the activity of Nature comes to a standstill as far as your particular soul is concerned.

So the result is a realised man, a soul which has realised its Being, its identity with the Divine — it cancels the cosmic existence. If one is active in the dynamic, he misses the static. If one remains in the static Brahman, one loses connection with the active dynamisation of the same Brahman. The solution is in the individual, the bridge between the passive and the active aspects of the Reality, between God and Nature, between the creator and the creation. The living bridge is man because he epitomises in himself the Divine.

If the Divine Reality contains both the aspects in itself — the passive and the active — so does man. There is a level where all is static, all is passive, silent; there are levels where there is movement, there is action, but they are not compartmentalised. There are walls of ignorance, certainly, which separate the one from the other, but as one takes steps to thin and then to dissolve these walls of separativity, it is realised that after all action takes place on the bosom of the Silence. It is a passive Reality which sustains and pours itself into the active manifestation.

It is in the measure in which man develops himself in a comprehensive way, combines in himself his awareness of the static Reality, and comprehends the various formulations in manifestation, in a word, the active Reality, that he proceeds and succeeds in embodying in himself the Divine Reality in manifestation.

*
* *
*

Last time I had occasion to mention to you about a mantra that Sri Aurobindo had given to Champaklal in the very beginning of his career here. This time I have brought the text of a message given by Mother to Champaklal on the first day of his work here. As you are all aware, he has been a worker with Mother and Sri Aurobindo during the last five decades without break, and he has been in certain ways a model for other workers. And this message that the Mother gave him, and which has sustained him all through, he was kind enough to share with me last week, and I thought you would be interested to hear it.

Here are the guidelines given by the Mother to an ideal worker whose name has become, in our Ashram, a byword for dedicated service to the Divine.

> Be simple.
> Be happy.
> Remain quiet.
> Do your work as well as you can.
> Keep yourself always open towards me.
> This is all that is asked from you.

Be your natural self. Do not load the mind with any sense of the importance of your role. Be just what you are — a child and servant of the Divine with such equipment as you have been given.

Be simple.

Do not tease yourself with notions of your inadequacies or fear of failure. After all the work is being done not by your capacities or powers but by the Divine Shakti to which you have to open yourself. Have trust in the Divine and do not torment yourself with complexes of inferiority or insufficiency.

Be happy.

Do not excite yourself and throw out your energies pell-mell. Effective work is done only when you are collected and calm within. Otherwise there is waste, the atmosphere is spoiled and the work suffers. Whatever circumstances, hold yourself in your poise.

Remain quiet.

Exert yourself quietly and to the best of your ability. Serve according to your best light. Deliberately summon all the faculties that are to participate in the work before you and put in your best. Remember the best of today prepares you for a greater best tomorrow. Be always at your peak.

Do your work as well as you can.

Do not be centred in yourself, in your abilities or your disabilities. The most you can do on your own is but a trifle and of little significance in yoga. What is important is that you should keep yourself open and receptive to the Divine, to the Higher Consciousness and Force that is to guide and embody itself in you. This is easier if you are fortunate in having a human embodiment of the Divine with whom you can enter into direct relation, to whom you can offer yourself and your work. You have the Mother who consents in her Grace and calls:

Keep yourself always open to me.

This is your part — simplicity without complications and artificialities of attitude and form; a cheerful spirit; quietude in poise and freedom from excitement in work; full exertion of yourself without lethargy and incomplete will; constant opening to the guiding light and effectuating Force of the Mother.

That is all that is asked from you.

All else will be done for you by the Divine to whom you leave all the results of your work, all the responsibilities of the situation, in love and joy.

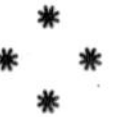

It was only two or three days ago that the Mother was explaining that falsehood is again and again falling upon her. And she said it is worse than physical torture. If it were physical torture, she could bear it, but this falling of falsehood continuously is more than she can bear.

She said that the difference in consciousness has become so much that every touch brings an ordeal. Her actual words were: "Falsehood is falling upon me again and again."

Whether she meant the falsehood in the world outside, the falsehood in the universe, or falsehood in the small world constituted by all of us is more than I can say. But I do feel it is the responsibility of each one to see that in his or her individual life there should be no falsehood. So that when we think of her and send our love to her in her present state it may reach her in its purity.

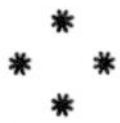

Sri Aurobindo's consciousness has always been fused in her, even as he lives in her atmosphere, in her. So her consciousness directs as before, as powerfully as ever. It is only her outer consciousness that is — I wouldn't say withdrawn — indrawn, but all things are still guided and directed by her. She is in touch, in her own way, with everything that goes on.

She asked someone last week, "How are things?" And he replied "Yes, everything is all right". Because he didn't want to give Mother all the details, he said everything was all right. Mother said, "You are saying everything is all right but I know things are not all right." Then she spoke to him saying that there is a good deal of disharmony in the atmosphere and that is delaying things. So, somehow, it is this disharmony that should be eliminated. She spoke to him for quite some time.

Can it be said that the active Brahman is the same as the Shakti Brahman or is there a difference?

Brahman as power is Shakti; Brahman can be realised as Power, as Consciousness, as Existence, as Bliss. So when you speak of Shakti, it is a power of the active Brahman.

No more difficulties of the mental being? So our next step is to go to the cosmic consciousness when we meet next.

12

Cosmic Consciousness

Cosmic consciousness is a loose term used with varying connotations in the world today. I have seen the term used for a feeling of universal sympathy, for expressing love for humanity — a sort of intense humanism. But the truth of cosmic consciousness is quite different.

Normally man is identified with his mind, life and body. When however he analyses his own consciousness or awareness, he comes to realise that he is not quite one with his mind, life and body, but that there is some meaning to it when he refers to "my life, my mind, my body". So he scrutinises the content of this mind and stumbles upon the "I" which is the pseudo-self with which he identifies himself. With a keener awareness, it doesn't take him long to realise that this "I" is only the ego-personality. Going still further, he steps into the region of the Self, the individual Self which is at the core of his personality.

Even that is not all. As he observes himself, he realises that even the individual Self is a derivation, is a representation of another Reality which transcends his own formula — let us call it the Transcendent. He sees that what he used to think as himself is only a semblance, an appearance of the Self that is within himself. And this Self, further, only represents in terrestrial terms the Reality that is Transcendent.

The individual Self and the Transcendent Reality do not exhaust life. There is around him the vast universe, the fantastic outpouring of a million-bodied Energy at different levels. When he analyses what the truth of that is, he gets a glimpse into the Truth of the universal extension. He feels, and he comes to recognise in due course, that even the universe around him has a reality which is at least as real — if not more real — as his own Self. He sets about understanding things, cognising the universal movement, and in the course of evolution he enlarges his consciousness and his vision to contact the universe at different points.

This extension of an individual consciousness to gradually identify itself with the universal consciousness spread in the universe is a psychological discipline which may be called "Yoga". There are yogas and yogas; there is a yoga of going within and finding the Reality within oneself; there is another line of yoga which pulls the individual consciousness upwards, crosses the various ranges of existence, and links it to the Transcendent Reality. There is another line by which one expands and enlarges one's being and embraces the universe in larger and larger segments.

To come back to the starting point, once we have the perception and the conception based upon it that the whole universe is a movement, we see the basis on which the whole movement turns. And there we come across the conception and the experience of the Self. Just as in the individual universe, in the individual movement, there is the base on which everything turns, — the individual Self — similarly in the universe too, there is the universal Self, a silent witness watching and holding the mighty movement of the universal forces.

If you realise this universal Self a little deeper, you will see that it supports the universal movement but is not involved in it. This very watching, this very regard of the Self, is a support to the movement.

Once you realise the universal Self upon which, in which the universal movement takes place, it leads you to the next step. You realise this Reality of the Self as the Lord and Master of the Universe. If the Reality first reveals itself as a detached, uninvolved witness, on a higher plane it assumes the status of mastery, of lordship. It is for delectation of that consciousness of the Lord that the universal nature plays out its universe. It is because the Lord has something to manifest out of his oceanic being that his own power, the universal Shakti is active.

This second realisation of the Divine as the Master and the Lord of the universe is a capital experience. It is that which gives a purpose and a direction to one's life. If one stops short at realising the Self as the only Reality, logically it follows that the world is either a mechanical movement or an illusion. But if you have patience enough and the Grace to guide you to realise the Divine in its aspect of the overlord, as the master of the universe, your vision opens into the dynamic reality of the Divine.

Indeed, when the mind first realises this aspect of the mastery and the lordship of the Divinity above, it is inclined to bifurcate the experience. It feels that there is a plane where the divine knowledge, the divine power reigns supreme but on the lower plane of the terrestrial universe the divine mastery is not absolute, it is truncated. So the mind believes in the superior reality of the upper hemisphere, and convicts the lower hemisphere of perpetual ignorance and falsehood. And the only logical issue is to escape from the lower into the higher. But this is so only when the mind stops halfway to its spiritual heights.

If it continues in its journey further, if it ascends in its consciousness, opening up the higher ranges of illumination, of will, of knowledge, it gets into the proper poise and sees that the universe is only He who has gone abroad. In the most ancient Upanishad — the Isha — the seer describes this in memorable terms. He says, "It is He that has gone abroad — that which is bright, bodiless, without scar of imperfection, without sin, pure, unpierced by evil — it is He who has gone abroad. The seer, the thinker, the one who becomes everywhere."

Mark the sequence, — first the poise of the seer. He sees,

what Sri Aurobindo describes in *The Life Divine*, the Real-Idea. When the Supreme is out to manifest, the Truth to be manifested is first seen as the seed idea. It holds, as if in a microfilm, all that is to come, all that is to unroll itself. He sees; He is the seer. After the seer, the next step is the thinker. What is seen is cogitated upon, given a spiritual substance. And then, the One becomes everywhere. After visualising, after brooding upon it, He delivers himself, unrolls himself— the One who becomes everywhere.

The Self-Existent has ordered objects perfectly according to their nature from years sempiternal. He has imposed his own order. If, to our petty eyes, blinded by limited vision, it looks disordered, it is not his fault. If, in the course of the yogic enlargement of consciousness one identifies oneself with that creative consciousness of the Lord, as it spreads itself, if one realises the Self as it becomes the Many,— not the static Self, but the dynamic Self — one knows that there is a perfect order. As Mother says, everything is as it should be at each moment. If it were not, the whole cosmos would fall to pieces. That is a design of providence in the course of evolution where a million possibilities are clashing. All possible care is taken by the intelligent eye to see that things are just what they should be.

When one realises that, one sees that the very experiences which provoke different reactions in the state of ignorance, evoke quite different responses in the state of Knowledge.

In the same Upanishad it is said, "He in whom it is the Self-Being that has become all existences that are the Becomings, for he has the perfect knowledge, how shall he be deluded, whence shall he have grief who sees everywhere oneness?" He has no grief, he has no pain, he has no suffering. He sees Truth as it is. Even what appears to us as pain, as weakness, as lack of power, he can see in its true perspective. He sees everywhere the play of Saccidananda, Existence-Consciousness-Bliss.

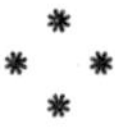

It is the Bliss which at times makes an impact more positively; at times it holds itself back from a consciousness which cannot stand it. Knowledge spreads itself, holds itself back. This holding back results in ignorance. He sees all as light and shade; he sees that there is no finality about the imperfections, about the drawbacks. He sees all is a play, and by adjusting one's own consciousness, one can participate in that manifestation of the Supreme.

In the yogic endeavour he raises himself to the heights of the spiritual mind, realises the Self in its dynamic aspect, and projects himself into the universe on the lower planes of existence and identifies himself with the becoming Transcendent Self as the Universal Existence. That is one way.

The second way that Sri Aurobindo describes to acquire this consciousness is not immediately to go above, but to expand laterally. One can have the realisation of Saccidananda on any plane of existence, because this higher triple principle is involved in each plane of existence. It is possible, by concentrating on the material plane of existence to realise the Divine on the physical level; so on the vital level, so on the mental level.

What the seeker does in this line of yoga is to accustom himself mentally to the idea of oneness, of love, of harmony, of universal joy. First the mind has to be educated and trained to breathe the atmosphere of oneness. Thereafter, he forces, or puts a pressure on his emotional being, on his heart to feel, to identify itself with larger and larger sections of humanity in the world. Simultaneously, he calls upon the higher power to descend into him, the higher consciousness to settle in him and release him from the limitations of the lower formula. And by this double pressure — outward and upward and calling down the divine Consciousness into oneself, there is a slow breaking of the walls so that the individual gradually assumes a larger and broader consciousness. The individual consciousness then has its moments of entering into the cosmic dimension. That is the beginning.

By persistent cultivation, by culture of the whole system in that dimension, one identifies oneself more and more completely with the cosmic or the universal consciousness. At every level — physical, vital, mental — one feels the oneness, one feels the impact of the universal matter, universal life, universal mind. In the process — at any rate in the beginning — the pains and griefs and sufferings of others make impacts upon one's being. Unfortunately, however, the joys and pleasures and bliss of other people don't make so much impact as the opposites do. That also is a stage, but that is not a stage to be indulged in. It happens only when the soul consents to stay on an inferior level of nature. Once it transcends the normal level of nature and detaches itself, it can receive the universal impacts. It does so not by participating in the suffering, not by participating in the pain and grief but with a certain measure of sympathy, understanding, and reaching out its help — the help of its strength, its love, its harmony.

As the endeavour proceeds, one rises above and is able to respond to the negative impacts — of pain, grief, suffering — by positive responses, not indifference, but positive, healing responses. One sees the play of the universal knowledge, the universal delight, the universal existence all over. Forms change, processes change, but the Reality continues to manifest. How far the individual consciousness remains separate from the universal consciousness so realised is another question.

It is possible for the individual consciousness to retain its individuality and at the same time have a constant relation in the play. It is also possible for it to look upon itself as a lower term, a smaller term of which the Universal Consciousness is a larger or higher term. But the truth of the matter is, both the individual and the universal are two terms of another reality, the Transcendental, the Supreme Saccidananda. The individual consciousness cannot get contact with this Supreme Saccidananda on its own plane except through the intermediary of the Truth-Consciousness plane — the Supermind, or the Supramental. It is there that both the upper and the lower hemispheres find their true meeting place; it is there that the One and the Many fuse together; it is there that knowledge and will, which are so separate on our plane, reveal themselves as two aspects of the same reality. It is only when man establishes connection between that plane of Truth-Knowledge and his own, that it is possible for him to break the walls between himself and the higher hemisphere of Saccidananda, and opens up his being entirely for the descent of the powers and principles of Truth, Will and Bliss in their entirety. This is the spiritual verity which has been described picturesquely in the ancient Veda as the eternal sacrifice wherein man offers the intoxicating wine of delight that he distils out of his life-experience to the gods and the gods descend in him setting up true harmony, a harmony of an orchestrated whole, opening up a new chapter in the Divine Manifestation.

It is a concept to those who are outside the realm of joy and pain, those who are aloof. But for those who are involved, it is much more than a concept — it is a fact of life. As long as the consciousness is at the level where pain and suffering impinge as realities, it will not be able to look beyond. It can do so only if at some point it can feel that the pain and suffering need not be there under certain conditions. If that enlightenment comes either by Grace or by experience and evolution, then pain itself becomes a concept, which is true under certain conditions but need not be true under other conditions.

So, ultimately, it depends upon the attitude of the

consciousness. And the attitude of the consciousness depends upon the stage of evolution at which it has arrived. If it has arrived at the possibility of leaping beyond the human level, then it sees that pain and misery are not the final term. Till one realises this and sees the possibility of translating it into one's own life, it is right and necessary that those who have experienced it should din that possibility into the ears of those who have not. And that is the role of scriptures, of practical philosophies which show the way. One is not expected just to read them and keep quiet; one has to follow them. But someone has to show the direction. So, even as a concept it has a value and it needs to be emphasised. To most, God is a concept; later one stumbles into a stage where it becomes a percept, and then it becomes a reality.

That is the process used by ethics — and a necessary process. First, I, the individual, feel "I am important"; gradually, as I grow, I include my family members. So to that extent my ego includes them for it stands to benefit by the welfare of the many around it. So in the process, my ego enlarges itself — I feel when somebody else suffers, I rejoice in their joy, I am concerned about their welfare. So it is not about myself alone, but about those around, the members of my family.

Then comes the immediate society, then the community, then the country, then the world — that way, in expanding circles, my ego goes on expanding itself, till one day it bursts. Once you realise mentally and feel emotionally that you are one with all humanity, all the petty things that weigh with you normally on an individual scale, don't move you afterwards. To that extent you are liberated from the individual bounds. So once you get accustomed to move in larger rounds, say for instance, of humanity, of the whole of mankind, or the whole of living creation, a little shock here or there, a little opening, becomes enough for you to be flooded with That which is around. Sri Aurobindo has said, that the

Divine is always on the lookout for those points which are ready — and when He finds them He just puts pressure on them. So the ultimate deliverance comes from a touch from above.

Desire, too, has to be plucked out in its different garbs. As we expand our consciousness, desire takes a correspondingly enlarged form. The desire to do good to myself, the desire to do good to my family, the desire to enrich my community, the desire to enrich my country at the cost of others — all these are but varying editions of desire. So it is not that desire can be plucked out once and for all; like the ego it has so many formations. Both desire and ego have to be scrutinised repeatedly and offered up to the Supreme Truth. Behind desire there is the truth of aspiration, desire is its deformation. The ego is a deformation, a shadow of the Self. The false formations, deviations have to go; the true entities have to emerge. At every step both desire and ego have to be eliminated.

An astrologer friend of mine came to see me in the last week of May. He always tells me things, even when I don't ask. He told me many glorious things about myself, then I asked him, "Why don't you tell me something about Mother?" I always ask him about Mother because in 1953 or 1954 — some twenty years ago — when Mother was going to the playground, playing tennis, meeting hundreds of people every day, distributing things twice, thrice and spending so much time with us — say from four in the morning to ten at night — he had said, a time was coming when Mother would stop coming to the playground. Thereafter she would confine herself to her room — she would meet people, but she herself won't come out. At that time everybody laughed at him. They said it was simply impossible, how could he say that? But he told it to Mother and Mother was very much interested in what she heard. His stock went up immediately and many people started consulting him. Then he told me once — he gives me every year a chart of what is going to happen in my spiritual life — :"During these months you are going to have a very devastating experience; it will be something like a spiritual death, but the Grace is there and you will pass through some transformation." I told Mother about it. She smiled and asked "What are the months he has told you?" And I replied "From October to December 10." "Let us see," she said. And then I forgot about it. Later on, she remembered — after the period was over — "Your astrologer friend had said something; what happened?" Then this gentleman told me, "Of course things may have happened and you may not have known."

He told me two or three weeks ago when he came for his vacation, that this period of stress — Mother was undergoing certain changes within herself — would change after June 10th. And today we are at June 6th; I think he is very near to the truth and if things continue at this rate things will be very bright after the 10th.

It is indicated in her horoscope, he said, that it will continue like this till the end of this year, but things will be brighter after the 10th June. We all know that neither Mother nor Sri Aurobindo nor for that matter any yogin can be determined by horoscopes and astrology; still he finds indications on the basis of his calculations. He said a very interesting thing which struck me profoundly. He said that the Mother's horoscope runs up to a hundred years only, thereafter it is left to the subject of the horoscope to determine its future course.

Doesn't Mother say in "Notes on the Way" that at every point it's a matter of choice between life and death?

Yes, she does. But this is from the astrological point of view. What she says is true, always, for her. But this — the horoscope does not stop there, do you follow me? It is a continuing horoscope, it doesn't stop. It is something unique.

13

Oneness

We are on the threshold of Oneness. We have seen how when we withdraw the concentration of our consciousness from the body, mind and life — on which it is normally fixed — and turn it inwards, we come to the status of our Self. Persisting in this, we perceive and realise the identity of this Self, deep within us, with an immutable Reality — what the Upanishads call the Brahman — at the back of all. And if we persist still further through this immutability, through this immobile reality, we pass into an impersonality that pursues us from the bounds of our personality. We enter the domain of the Transcendent Reality. It is possible that on the way, if our path is not too narrow, we may have the experience of the Cosmic Consciousness, the consciousness of the universe around us. We may also realise the Divine as the Lord of the universe. But these are all experiences on the path, circumstances that one passes through, but the goal is always transcendence in impersonality, in silence.

This is the goal of the traditional path of knowledge, but that is not all. Sri Aurobindo points out that, having reached the status of transcendence, it is possible to turn back and, through the cosmic consciousness, realise also the One Reality in its multitudinous aspects. Not only realise the Brahman in his immobile status, but also in his variegated mobility of status and movement.

The seeker of the integral knowledge pursues this path. He realises the Saccidananda, the Reality of Existence, Consciousness and Bliss, in its unity on every level; but unity coterminous with the diversification of that unity into multiplici At every stage he realises this Existence as one and many; this Consciousness-Force as originally one, but throwing itself out to multiply; one Delight streaming into varied currents of joy and delight. It is when he holds to this conception of Saccidananda on every plane, that he doesn't lose his grip over the manifestation.

Sri Aurobindo describes how the seeker of the Integral Path of Knowledge realises in his own being, on the seven planes of creation — which are reproduced in himself, — this truth of Saccidananda. He first realises that there is a sheer Existence, an Absolute which is not touched by anything that goes out or comes back. It is always there; whatever else may be or may not be there, there is this Existence — one Soul. On every plane there is this reality at the back.

On its own plane of existence — the highest — the seeker who has the realisation also views the spread-out of this Existence, the spread-out of this Unity into a multiple unity. This multiple unity is not arrived at by totalling up all that you see into one total. The Reality is everywhere; wherever you look, you see that it is the same Reality — that is why it is called 'One'. Essentially, the one existence is everywhere. Similarly, the consciousness and the force of that consciousness, though essentially one, are thrown out, self-diversified into a million energies, into a million thought-forces, but all deriving from the one original Chit. So too, the one delight, the ocean of bliss that is one, underneath all creation, throws out so many jets, so many waves of its currents which we call, according to our capacity of receiving it or not being able to receive it in ourselves, as joy or sorrow, pleasure or pain. When, by discipline, we are able to enlarge our consciousness, the base of our consciousness, and can receive, can embrace the waves of delight that come upon us fully, there is no more pain. So the first step to eliminate pain and suffering is to enlarge ourselves, to break out of the walls of our division which are erected by our ego.

After Delight, there is the Truth-Mind, the Truth-

Principle, which is always in possession of the one Truth, but directing so many flames from the one fire of Truth, launching each one on its career, but always with the background of that Unity.

Then there is the mind, the mind gradation of Saccidananda, where all is one consciousness at the mental level. This is parcelled out, apparently, in a million minds. But in spite of the number it is one mind. So, too, with the life-force, which is fragmented into so many forms, each of which insists on being separate from the others. And then there is universal matter out of which all forms are shaped, and to which they all go back when they are broken.

These are the seven gradations of Saccidananda which the seeker of the integral knowledge has to realise. Not only must he realise in his experience, in his consciousness, but he has to build up a vision in which he sees every movement of life, every form of life, every experience of life in terms of this unity of Saccidananda.

There is also another aspect. There are what are called the upper and the lower hemispheres of existence. In the upper belt, that of Saccidananda proper, the Saccidananda is unveiled, is revealed to experience. But in the lower hemisphere it is veiled. What we call the organisation of mind is really a projection of the consciousness aspect of Saccidananda. But the consciousness aspect is held back, is veiled by the fragmented formation of mentality. Similarly, the life-force, the life-world, is a projection, again, of the force of the consciousness above — the Tapas — which, because of fragmentation of division confesses to a certain impotence, disintegration, and does not manifest the omnipotence of the original Consciousness-Force. So also matter is the sensible mould of the spirit; as Sri Aurobindo describes it, it is the "robe of the spirit". If the spirit is concealed, that is because there is the veil and the cloud of ignorance.

As the yoga of knowledge proceeds, one begins to link the

upper and the lower hemispheres, realise the higher Truth as expressed in the lower terms, in however deformed a manner. But even the best of us, as long as we stand on the summits of the mind, work under a certain handicap and we can never have the full figure of the Saccidananda reflected below. It is only when we open our consciousness to the intermediate link of the Supramental consciousness, the Supermind, or the Truth-mind, that the gulf begins to be healed. The Higher Reality, in its integrality begins to communicate itself to the lower intelligence through the Truth-mind.

The Veda describes how, when man rises to the level of this brilliantly lit mind, the luminous mind of the sun, seven rivers flow down. They are the rivers of inspiration, illumination, intuition, and many other kinds, which reveal their character to the practitioner of yoga. It is only when this downpour from the Supramental consciousness is effected that the gulf between the lower and the higher hemisphere begins to close, and we have truly one perspective, one unbroken gradation from the depth of insentient matter to the heights of the supernal Existence-Consciousness-Bliss.

This, then, is the process of the Integral yoga of knowledge — not the traditional yoga of knowledge, mind you. In its process, in its working, you will see that the goals of the three traditional paths of knowledge, of work, of love, are fulfilled. For the yoga of knowledge aims at knowing the truth of existence; what after all is true, what is the true nature of one's own existence? The Integral yoga of knowledge first gives you the realisation, "I am not different, I am not other than He who is the Saccidananda". This is declared in the famous formula "He am I" (*So'ham*). When this realisation is attained, there is a unique oneness between myself and Him who pervades and transcends all creation.

As a consequence, I also see Him not only in unity with myself, but in unity with all around me. I realise my oneness not only with the Saccidananda purusha, but with the cosmic purusha as well. My union with Him is fulfilled in my union with Him in other forms. I realise the Lord of Existence, the Lord of the Universe, whose will pervades and controls all the movements. And, once having perceived that will of the Master, — Master of my existence and Master of a million existences around — my will tunes itself to that Will. I cease to work for my salvation; I cease to work for the salvation of others as well. But I work to fulfill that master Will of which, I begin to see, my own will is a tiny projection. This is the grand aim of the yoga of works.

And having realised the Reality as a Supreme Person above and behind the universe, as the Lord of the universe, within the cosmos, I also perceive Him in His aspect of Delight, of Bliss, which expresses itself in the universe as the fount of Love. After all, Love is an expression taken by Bliss. Bliss wants to enjoy itself — it posits itself in one form, takes another form and bridges them — and this interchange and love, swallowing up of one Bliss by another Bliss, one form of Bliss by another form, is Love, fusion, union. This realisation of the Love aspect and the bliss aspect of Saccidananda is the grand aim of the yoga of devotion.

These three ends are successively fulfilled by the successful practice of the Yoga of integral knowledge. To one who has arrived at this crown of achievement, there are no human problems. As the Upanishad says, "How shall he grieve, what problems can he have who sees everywhere oneness?" Problems arise when there is a second; fear arises when there is another. When you see all as one, there is no room for any problem. This is the theme of oneness.

Before we start yoga, we must have a mental appreciation of this truth of oneness. As we proceed, we must always remember this oneness and recall it to our mind whenever we are threatened with division in our own consciousness, division with others and a feeling of being 'left out'. And the traditional means to practise, to make real to ourselves this sense and truth of oneness is the celebrated mantra that is known as OM.

It was only last week that I was given the text of a letter written by a devotee to Mother some years ago. He had written, "It often occurs to me to beg thee for a key word for japa". The Mother gave OM and that was no surprise, for the Mother has always attached a special importance to this word of words, and there was a time when she was daily repeating it audibly in her chamber. I remember this particularly because she had explained at that time how the word is to be pronounced. Most people accent the first syllable and the last peters out. The Mother pointed out that all the syllables are to be clearly and fully articulated, and especially the last 'mm' should be rounded up with amplitude and clarity. I tried it and found a difference in the vibrations set up when the 'mm' is left half-enunciated, or swallowed up, and when it is pronounced clearly. Most people in their hurry to repeat the mantra a hundred times, two hundred times, or as often as they have decided, go on saying 'om, om, om' as if it is a chore that must be quickly finished.

Any questions?

The last time you talked about widening of consciousness. I'd like to get a better idea of what you mean by that term . . .

At the level where I am aware I begin by extending my emotions, my feelings to embrace not merely my own interests, but the interests of those around me. After some time, the interests of those who are not connected with me but are still there are also included for they also are manifestations of God. Similarly, the area in which my mental thoughts move has to be gradually and wilfully extended to cover broader and broader areas so that there is a continuous, ceaseless effort on the conscious levels of my being to leave my ego-centred self and expand myself, identify myself with larger and larger circles of humanity. Side by side, I recognise that beyond what is perceptible, beyond what is sensible to me, there are other realms of consciousness and being and I consciously try to open out into those regions of consciousness. This effort which starts mentally, gradually creates certain grooves in nature by which all movements tend to flow into broader currents. The idea is to broaden my ego more and more till the "island ego joins its continent."

Would you also become sensitive to what is around you by that process?

Yes, definitely. Sri Aurobindo describes in his chapter on the "Cosmic Consciousness", that the heart beats in unison with the heartbeats of all. Their vibrations of joy and suffering fall on you. But that is only the first step; to suffer the sufferings of others is only the first step. As one rises above, one can understand, take note of the sufferings of others without oneself suffering them. One can also give a healing touch. From his higher position, one can direct waves of understanding, waves of sympathy that will help one's suffering brothers. The identification is complete. At times it is very inconvenient also because even the thoughts of others echo in the corridors of one's mind. But they're all stages, and if one persists the path forms itself.

Then as one gradually becomes aware, the periphery becomes less defined; the ego separates. Would you say one is dissolved ultimately?

The ego is certainly dissolved at a certain stage in this expansion of consciousness, but the psychic center remains. It becomes strong, it becomes active as a point for the radiation of the Infinity, for the functioning, from a particular point of the Light. The center continues, in the oceanic being of the cosmic person, but it is an individuality without walls, it is so to say a sort of pin-point for a particular stress of consciousness and expression.

I was trying to separate an egoistic wideness from the sense of Infinite wideness that comes when you experience the higher realms.

After a certain stage the ego thins out, unless one perversely stays at the vital level and like Hitler, like Stalin, becomes a center of vital ego of domination; that is a deformation. The seeker knows and he is always alert to cast out the shadows of the vital. So there can also be a mental ego, a colossal mental ego that feels, for instance, that its philosophy is the only salvation, and it insists on imposing it on every mind. The ego has many personalities. It is only if the psychic is awakened that the ego does not get the scope to posture, to pose as the true Divine.

In an actual work, like the building of the Matrimandir, which demands for all of us engaged in it the manifesting of protection as we work, how can a harmony be achieved when there are varying levels of consciousness at work on it, particularly the core of it – it is designing and structuring. How can that harmony be achieved when there are these various levels and the work has its own momentum?

In such a dynamic situation, there can never be a total and a final harmony at any stage. Because so many elements are involved, each at its own level of consciousness. Mother says that if each one, at any rate, among those who are awakened, takes care to function at the highest level of consciousness one has attained, there is generated a certain force of goodwill which breaks down the element of friction. Each one functions at his best and highest, and even if he knows that what he has is the right solution, he will not impose it on others who are unwilling to accept it. He will have an understanding of the inability of others to fall in, so he accepts, for the time being, the consensus that is arrived at or that is possible at the moment, but goes on exerting a silent pressure — in all humility — from within on the situation. You exert from your level, I exert from my level, but ultimately if the exertion of our will is free from ego, from wanting to prove it right and others wrong, it does create a movement, in a subtle way, in the right direction and something happens to convince the others that they are not going the right way. Or those obstructing elements are removed from the scene; but in no case should the work be hampered.

One can always try with the means at one's disposal to convert others to one's own point of view, but should one fail, one should not sulk and deny his cooperation. In a collective effort one has to carry on with as many people as possible. That is why success in a collective effort is always more difficult. The general level of life is lower than the individual level.

If the work suffers, or is allowed to suffer, as a result of such a situation, we have to take it as the way of the working of the higher will. Work is not an end in itself; work is a field for the growth of consciousness. You grow by doing the work well, another person grows by committing faults; the way of growth for each is not the same.

Mother said, I remember, to this effect: "Be at the height of your consciousness, find out the area of agreement with others, station yourself there and try to extend that area."

14

The Soul and Nature

It is the province of integral knowledge to gather together all the elements of existence, individual and collective, and find their unity in their common Absolute. The Divine, when it manifests, holds in itself the absolute term of everything that issues from it, and when we approach from our end, for every faculty, every part, there is a larger term in the universe, and an absolute of both in the Divine. So it is in the process of working out the scheme of integral knowledge that the whole of the universe comes to be embraced; nothing is left out. It is true for a certain approach of the mind, that the absolute of everything is only to be found in the Beyond. In time and space there cannot be an Absolute; everything is limited. It is above this universe that you find the Absolute.

In a sense, Sri Aurobindo points out, this is true. But it is also true that the Absolute does not forfeit its character just because it pours itself out in terms of the individual and the cosmic. All the principles of existence are present in the universe at all levels. The principle of absoluteness also is present, in principle, everywhere.

For instance, let us take the principle of Soul and Nature; this is an ancient institution of duality, conceived and pictured differently by different systems of religion and philosophy. There are some schools which speak of the soul as the Self and Nature as the power of the Self covering Itself with any number of illusions. Why the Self should choose to cover itself with illusions instead of truths, no system has been able to say. However, there are other schools which consider the Self as the Being and Nature as the power of that Being to formulate itself in innumerable forms and movements.

There is also, as we have seen in one of our earlier discussions, the duality of Ishwara, the Lord and his Shakti, his puissance. He is not only the Lord, the Self that stands behind, but he is also the Master and the Power that issues from him; the Power that builds, does so for his delectation.

In the ancient Indian systems there is what is called the Sankhya system which many of you must have come across in Sri Aurobindo's *Essays on the Gita.* The Sankhya derives its name from the Sanskrit term for "enumeration". Its basic principle is the enumeration of the twenty-five principles that constitute existence. It conceives of an uninvolved Soul, Self facing Nature. Nature and Soul are eternally separate and distinct. Nature goes into movement, the Self regards it and Nature goes on playing, building, withdrawing, all for the pleasure or the benefit of the Soul. These souls are multiple, but Nature is one. As long as the Soul looks at Nature, whom Sri Aurobindo describes somewhere else as the nautch girl, the dancer who enacts the play of the cosmos for the pleasure of the Self or the Soul, the movement continues. The moment the witnessing Soul withdraws his gaze the impulse stops; Nature comes to a standstill.

The Sankhyans were very clever. If they had conceived of one Soul, then the moment one person achieved this withdrawal, and nature stopped her play, it would be repeated in everyone. That is why they said there are innumerable souls, multiple souls watching the play of one Nature taking her position vis-a-vis each different soul.

Now these are some of the main ways of presenting the problem of the duality, Soul and Nature. This duality, Sri Aurobindo points out, starts from the very summits of creation, and it reproduces itself on every level. In the *Essays on the Gita* this relation between the Soul and Nature is graphically described, step by step, keeping with the growth, the progress of the evolutionary movement. First is the Soul as the witness; it does not participate in the play of Nature, but it just regards. No doubt, the very act of regarding is, in a sense, participation. If the Soul were not to witness, there would be no impulsion to Nature to continue her play.

However, even in this witnessing action of the Soul there are grades and grades. There is the tamasic witness that just watches without movement, without an effort to influence, or even to transcend and get away from the play. It just bears it, suffers it. Next there is what is called the rajasic witness, where the Soul regards not out of helplessness, but with a certain acute interest. There is also the regard of the sattwic type, where the Soul has attained a certain maturity and regards things with a tranquility of spirit. But the ideal witness, Sri Aurobindo points out, is he who looks on like a spectator regarding a play on the stage, drawing the full enjoyment of it, participating in his own emotions, but ready at any moment to walk off without being involved in it. This is the highest poise of the witnessing Soul as far as Nature is concerned.

The second poise is the poise of the sanctioner. The very act of witnessing implies a certain kind of implied sanction, indirect sanction. But in this next step the Soul exerts itself and makes a movement of affirming the impulsion of Nature, or holding it back, but without involving in subsequent activities. Once the Soul starts sanctioning, it is only a question of another step before he participates in the movement of Nature and constitutes himself as the controller; he controls, he directs the movement of Nature as he wishes. And this action of controlling and directing Nature by the Soul culminates, at its highest, in the Soul becoming the enlightened enjoyer of Nature. He is not helplessly subject to Nature, getting whatever few crumbs of enjoyment she throws at him, but is a fully conscious, enlightened enjoyer — that is the final step of the Soul as far as Nature is concerned.

All these steps, Sri Aurobindo points out, derive from the eternal duality that is in Saccidananda. Sat, Existence, is also the Existent — it's not merely an impersonal state, but it is a positive being whom you can't describe except to say that He exists. His consciousness, knowledge — Chit — and that Chit as consciousness-force, is the prototype of what projects itself as Nature in our terrestrial creation. It is the same ancient Puissance from the Lord that becomes, when it devolves into ignorance, what we call Prakriti. If the Purusha is still on the heights of his Self, or in the inmost depths, he still retains a link with the Divinity from which He has issued. So also Prakriti, Nature, is in her inmost depths, the Divine Consciousness-Power. It was of her that the ancient Upanishads spoke when they pointed out that the Rishis in their meditation discovered that She is the Puissance that is covered up in the modes of her working. What is called "Shakti" in knowledge, is "Prakriti" in ignorance. Just as the human soul in the belt of ignorance is subject to the law of nature and is ruled by nature, similarly the power of the soul, as long as the soul is in ignorance, is also subject to the colour of ignorance. The way out of this stigmata is first for the individual to become conscious in himself of the various parts of his being: his mind, his life-force, his soul, his physical body. After becoming conscious he has to find their link and correspondence with the universal Mind, the universal Life-Force, the universal Soul and the universal Matter. Naturally you start at the level of the mind, then come to the level of the senses — you sense it, you feel it — but before you can either know or sense, you have to have the vision. That vision you get by reading the books of those who have had that vision, or the vision simply dawns on you by Grace.

After the vision is real to you, it is translated in terms of the intellect as knowledge. From the level of the mind, you gradually render it in terms of feeling and experience, feel your oneness with the universal terms, find yourself in the cosmic being — that is, ultimately, the purpose of meditation, concentration which are periods when you get away from yourself, as Sri Aurobindo describes in Savitri:

> In moments when the inner lamps are lit
> And the life's cherished guests are left outside,
> Our spirit sits alone and speaks to its gulfs.

You find unknown and unseen faculties coming up, finding their link with their corresponding members in the cosmos.

But that is not the end, that is again only a stage. There is no attainment only by extending and universalising yourself for you still universalise yourself in ignorance. You are still within the boundaries of the shadow of ignorance. That is why Sri Aurobindo insists that simultaneously, or perhaps even before this step of extending and widening yourself horizontally is undertaken, you awake to the Divinity in you, link yourself with it, throw a hook to the Divine above, recover your original relation with the parent Divine, turn your will to be in tune with the Divine Will. When you are ready, when you have begun to function as a center of the Divine in the human form, then it is safe for you to extend yourself, identify yourself, and emerge as the cosmic man. Otherwise if you miss that verity, that truth within yourself, you are only undergoing the risk of colossalising your ego. One may feel vast, one may identify oneself with the larger mind or life-force, but if it is the mind poised in the ego, the life-force dominated by the ego, then it is a titanic or an asuric development that takes place — almost suicidal.

This, then, is the precaution. First an individual, psychic realisation, attunement to the Divine Will within yourself. In that consciousness, in that poise, you can safely extend yourself gradually and become one with the cosmic being.

Coming to questions, there is a question of a very practical type that confronts a seeker or an awakened person in the course of yoga. It is this: you begin to realise a certain falsity in your being, a certain limitation which besets your functioning. You find it is almost constitutional with you, chronic. Normally in the outside world one doesn't realise it. One always attributes failures, mistakes, to others, so the question does not arise. But once one steps into yoga there is no respite; one is not allowed to have that comforting delusion. Say you realise your handicap, your failing, then how do you set about correcting the situation? This situation arises in the lives of most of us at some time or other. We try, we fail. Now if we fail half a dozen times, is it an indication that things will remain always thus, that we will have to bear that cross all our life?

Well, a yogin cannot take up that attitude. When you take to the path of the Divine, the Mother has pointed this out repeatedly, every little thing that takes place in your life has a meaning. You have to keep your eyes open and your mind vigilant to discover what is its purpose, why it has happened. Now when the knowledge comes to you that you have a certain failing and you have to remedy it, it means that Nature has brought you to the first step of remedying the situation. The first step is always to become aware of the difficulty. And in truth, in the realm of Truth — whatever it may be in ignorance — knowledge always carries with it the necessary power to effectuate itself.

The bane of our creation in ignorance is this division between knowledge and power. It is only at the Truth-Consciousness level that Knowledge and Power reveal themselves as two sides of the same Reality — Knowledge is instinct with Power, Power is guided by Knowledge.

To continue, the very fact that you awake to the knowledge of your defect, your failing, guarantees that behind that awareness the necessary power is waiting to be drawn upon to translate that knowledge into practice. Nature always carries the means of effectuating the knowledge that it gives. In any field, the moment you have the perception, be sure that the means to translate the perception into practice is there. We may not realise it and in our wrong way of setting about things we may miss it, but it is there. With that faith that the reserves of the power required to deal with the situation are given to you — or will be revealed to you in due time — you set about correcting yourself. At every little situation you exert your will. You cannot say that you will do it on more important occasions and not in small matters. Every occasion should be taken to exert the will in the right direction, to summon all the energies, to remedy the situation as far as the circumstances permit. Once, twice, thrice, a hundred times the will has to be exercised, and the resistance is bound to give way; the power to remedy it is bound to grow.

It is very hard to see the Soul and Nature as a duality. In reading the chapter it seems Sri Aurobindo links it up into one line.

At a higher level of consciousness, Soul and Nature reveal themselves as one Reality. But the moment the stage of manifestation arrives, there is a polarity. The same reality poises itself doubly — Soul and Nature, the Master and the Power. Without these two terms — the same Reality, the same being positing itself doubly — there is no creation, there is no manifestation. In the Tantras it is said that in the beginning there is only one, the *Parashiva* the supreme Shiva. When he gets into the mood to create he poises himself as Shiva and Shakti. As you ascend, if once you decide "enough of this play, enough of this creation", then through the two gates you pass into the Supreme Absolute.

So far as the manifestation is concerned, there is a practical duality though essentially it is not so; the two are one just as sun and sunlight, fire and heat. For practical purposes we have to accept this working relation of duality.

There came to the Centre a message or rather a vision that Mother had on darshan day in November 1965. This was given by Mother to Rijuta to send to American centers in March, the month before she went into retirement. It was evidently given with her foreknowledge that this was to be a directive when she went into retirement, and it contains something very important for those who are engaged in an active karmayoga and at the same time who want to do the yoga of transformation, which she says was shown to her in the vision as being done by only a few. The essence of the vision was that Sri Aurobindo showed Mother the order within the universe, every being having its particular plane and said that there was no need to go out and change those who were contented with the light of a higher culture, with a harmony on the mental plane, because they were satisfied with the plane of consciousness on which they moved; to disturb that would not be right. If one is to do the yoga of transformation he must do it in his place, at his own level.

It is true, what you said. Mother was shown many gradations of humanity among which there was one special gradation which had reached the acme of human development, mental culture, had even shed the last elements of animality, but was content with the highest possible mental development. It had no special seeking for transformation and divinisation. But there were others; when Mother saw the different gradations — different kinds of people, different stages of evolution fitting in with different orders — she smiled at the idea of preparing people. She said only those who were ready and sought for a particular truth, would get it. There must be the aspiration and those who do not have it should be left to their state — am I right? They should be left to their state. Then she describes that there are some who are actively engaged in the yoga of transformation, they are working for it. There are also those who are contributing to the yoga of transformation in their way, without doing the yoga itself — by way of work, by way of goodwill, by helping in many ways. They themselves do not expect to participate in the gains of transformation; they know they are not fit for it but all the same they are putting in their best. They are doing their karmayoga and contributing to it. So each category must respect the other categories; they must not impose their discipline, their standards of sacrifice on the others. Each category must be left free to develop in its own way.

Mother says it is no use compelling a person to shed his animality when he is not ready for it. If he is still in the evolutionary stage which is proper to the animal belt, it's no use compelling him to desist from certain actions which are natural to the animal stage. If we are to follow only the gradations hewn by Nature at her pace it will take a long time to evolve. But man is given a will, man can expedite his evolution, man can take a leap. So if I find that certain parts in me still respond to the urges of animality, but there are other parts which aspire higher, which want to cross the belt, certainly, I am expected to exert my will and forcibly eliminate the inferior elements from my nature and catch up with the higher planes. Each sincere person is expected to do it and he is given the help to do it. All that is expected is that he shall not impose it on another person. But each individual has a certain responsibility when he is given the opportunity.

Yes, but in a community such as the one at Matrimandir there is a different set of conditions – it's the only settlement in Auroville that has a list of rules sent out with Mother's blessings for no sex indulgence, no tobacco, drugs, and so forth. Now when Mother's expressed wishes in these matters are not followed and when Mother has also said in reference to these injunctions, that her help is available to any sincere person who wants to change, what should be the attitude of a member of the community towards this?

The very fact that Mother has framed these guidelines for those who stay in Matrimandir, and she chooses certain individuals alone to stay there, necessarily means that they are in a stage when they can and should follow these guidelines. Otherwise they forfeit the trust imposed in them by the Divine. It is the responsibility of each one to respond and follow up, otherwise the trust is betrayed. I have seen how she makes the selection. Her method of selecting persons to stay here is different from the method used for other communities in Auroville. No individual has the right to interfere with the course of life of another unless it cuts across the discipline of the community. Individual lives are separate but there is an area where the collective life starts. There things are different and a pressure can be exerted at that level. Either an opinion must be created, a powerful opinion making it difficult for the offending elements to continue or it must be brought to the notice of Mother to see whether she will allow the situation to continue or not. Each individual has a certain responsibility to the collectivity here. The remark that one cannot compel another doesn't hold good here, in that vision. It does not apply here, because this is a select community, a sort of vanguard which cannot be permitted to slide back.

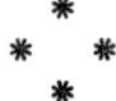

Power is originally Divine; as Love is Divine, Light is Divine, Power is Divine. It is only its perverted reflection in ignorance that becomes an energy of falsehood. Essentially, intrinsically, power is Divine. Possibly the seat of power in man, in a human being, is the vital, and the vital happens to be the most recalcitrant and aboriginal member of the human family. But as Sri Aurobindo has observed, the vital enlightened, the vital converted, is a hero of God, a soldier of the Divine. Without the vital falling in line there is no manifestation. Mother has laid so much stress on the conversion of the vital because the whole endeavour to bring the kingdom of heaven on earth is to be fed and supported by the complete participation of the vital which is the vehicle of power. Simply because in its present stage the vital happens to be primitive, you cannot convict it of eternal aboriginality. Power is neither moral nor immoral. It depends upon who uses it and why. Like electricity you can use it for a good and peaceful purpose or you can use it for a wrong purpose. Power is amoral. As Sri Aurobindo observes in that classic book

The Mother, Power, Money, Sex are the three Divine Puissances which have been misused. Power is Divine originally, we have to reclaim it for the Divine.

Can the leap for the transformation be effectuated on aesthetic levels?

Yes, but it will be confined to the aesthetic sphere. On that level it will be there, you will be linked. The value there will be different, the appreciation there will be different, but the rest of the being cannot share that attainment unless it is related dynamically to it. Many poets, seers, rishis have had this kind of transmutation on their high levels but they were not able to make it part of life on the whole. The artist, the painter, the musician at their summit do undergo a transmutation, they do break through the human horizons, and that is how they bring to the earth some glory from the heaven.

With her withdrawal isn't the Mother teaching us how to walk by ourselves in her consciousness? And how can a matter be referred to her without disturbing the state that she wishes to be in?

This withdrawal is temporary and, as you said, the presiding force is making use of this period to force people to feel the presence, force them to contact the central Reality and govern themselves without being guided at every step. We have to wait. There are signs already of her resuming effective control of the work. She said, only a couple of days ago, that she has been following an inner movement and she has arrived somewhere. The pressure is growing in a way that physical reference of things to her may not be found necessary at all.

I'd like to ask a question which concerns work and the position of those persons whose own feelings of the truth of what they ought to do does not coincide with what is laid down by someone who's directly appointed by the Mother as their superior. What should be done in this situation?

In the first place, we must assume the bonafides of both

the parties. The person who decides, executes must recognise the bonafides of those who differ from him. And the rest also must accept that the person in charge is doing things with the best of his light. That's the best he can do. We may not agree with it, we may not think it's the right thing, but it's the best he can do — we must accept that.

Now when the question arises of difference, we must be frank enough to put it to the person that we feel differently. If it is not possible at that time to put it before the Mother, we have the right to express our reservation, but still we must do what the person in charge asks to do; without this no collective work can go on. If there are a hundred individuals, there will be ninety opinions. We must have faith in the guiding power; all things ultimately fall into their proper position.

If the person in charge continues to do things really detrimentally to the interest of the work, you can trust to the guiding Grace to effect the necessary change in the right time. When she puts somebody in charge, Mother always puts a force in the person to guide him, to guard him from error, to help him. She also puts a force to evoke that amount of loyalty from others which is necessary. How he uses that power is another question. In these matters, ultimately, it is a question of everybody's sincerity. A very thin line separates the question of rightness and wrongness. Whether it is my ego that feels hurt and finds justification because my opinion is not accepted or whether it is the right thing that has been revealed to me and the other fails to appreciate it, it is very difficult to decide. It is only the utmost honesty with oneself that can help.

15

The Soul and its Liberation

We were discussing last time the relation between soul and nature, on the individual as well as on the universal level. We saw that on each plane this relation of soul to nature differs, and the state of consciousness one has at a moment depends upon the poise of the soul regarding its nature at that moment. Considered from any point of view, this is the crux of the matter: what exactly is the relation that obtains between soul and nature? Is the soul a subject, either a willing subject or a helpless subject to Nature? Or is the soul standing behind as a witness, perhaps taking note, but not interfering? Or is it that the soul rejects Nature, turns its gaze elsewhere? Or does the soul, after detaching itself in the first instance from Nature, thereafter assume mastery over Nature? Does it control and make Nature its own instrument? These are the various alternative relations possible between soul and Nature. According to the particular relation we accept, will be our outlook on life, our philosophy of life.

We have seen Sri Aurobindo's approach, how in his integral view all possible relations are worked out, step by step, as so many gradations in the evolution of the soul godwards. Once we accept this ideal, it goes without saying that the goal of our yoga ceases to be what it has traditionally been so far. We are no longer satisfied to allow the earth-life to live as it is lived around the ego. Neither are we satisfied in turning our back on earth, on the life on earth, and stepping into some beyond, leaving the earth as it is. Our aim is rather to reproduce in ourselves that standing relation which the

Divine Soul, which the Divine Being has with its Nature, in working out this manifestation. Not liberation, not escape, but a fulfillment of the Divine Soul whose intention it is to manifest the glory of the Divine through the workings of its own active force, which we call Nature, is our objective.

The starting point in the yoga of knowledge and the immediate goal is to arrive at the basic oneness which underlies all working in multiplicity. In the life around us we see many vicissitudes, many variations, many confusions — what Sri Aurobindo calls 'perversions of relations' — all of them are deformations, malformations of this basic unity. There is oneness in the Divine. Its active force of Delight, in the course of working out its urge to manifest, passes through several phases — incomplete, half-complete, more-or-less-complete — and according to the stage through which Nature is passing, there are these variations in the states of being, states of consciousness. Once, by discipline, by self-observation, by going behind the exterior surface and directing our gaze behind the veil, we discover that there is a unity of existence, there is a oneness of being, all things fall into their proper perspective.

This oneness, this effort of rediscovering oneness in the midst of multitude is to be brought about by the individual. No doubt the universal is a larger term, the transcendent Divine is still larger, but the working out of this process of manifestation, of the relation of Nature and soul, is done in the individual. The nodus of ignorance is certainly in the individual, at the point of his ego. But it is also due to this nodus in the individual that all movement towards progress starts. It is at the level of ignorance, at the level of the ego and desire that the movement of progression starts. It changes its character as we leave behind the original, impelling causes. The soul comes into its own gradually, but the person who has to work it out is the individual. In the world of ignorance, in the formula of ego and desire, it is the individual who bears the brunt of pain, evil and suffering. As he rises higher, as the scale of evolution builds up, it is again the individual who has to aspire, who has to receive the higher charge and work out in himself a developing relation of freedom, power and joy with Nature. He begins to realise, as he progresses, that Nature is not something alien of which he is a bond-slave. He realises that Nature is the force of his own soul, it is an active energy that has taken shape to do his bidding. If only he becomes conscious of his Self, of his real status in the soul, he gets freedom from Nature.

To get freedom from Nature, then, is the first objective and to get that freedom, detachment is the first step. In the midst of life, in the midst of movement, hold yourself back for a moment. Immediately you will become aware — may be for a moment, may be for a few minutes — of a gulf between your status of observation and the movement of Nature which goes on unconcerned whether you participate in it or not. This withdrawal now and then has to be gradually developed into an attitude of detachment. As this poise of detachment is repeated again and again, it gets established in the being, there is a spontaneous going back to that posture of detachment; there is a bifurcation between Nature and soul, Nature and oneself.

With the ascetic this detachment is allowed to develop into a divorce, but this way is not open to the seeker of the integral yoga. He has to gather up the strength, gather up the consciousness that grows in him out of detachment, and assume mastery over Nature. Once he assumes this mastery, he is in a position to manifest the Divine without interference, without deformation, without perversion. The individual continues to be the agent for the manifestation, for working out the fulfillment in the cosmos, not in the cosmos alone but also beyond it. Even in traditional yogas which don't admit the ultimate reality of the work and a purpose in life, in states of *samadhi* or trance — utmost concentration — it is the individual consciousness that looks up to the larger term of itself, the Transcendent Consciousness, the Absolute Brahman, and seeks to merge in it. Even there it is the individual soul which seeks to affirm its freedom from Nature, its freedom from all terms of manifestation — what it calls ignorance — and arrive at a merger in the Absolute. May be the Absolute is a Non-Being, what is called the Non-Existent of the Buddhists, or the sole Brahman of the Adwaita. Whichever the course chosen, the positive or the negative, the effect is a denial of the cosmos, which certainly is not the sole possible solution.

For the seeker of integral knowledge, every step has to be related to three terms: God, Nature, Individual. Once the individual comes into his own, he has next to re-form his relation with the world around; with the people around, with the movements around, with all the many tiers of creation around. He has to reset the relations, he has to approach them from the new angle of consciousness that he has realised. He has also to keep alive the relation with the Divine, that he has realised, constantly on the inner levels of his being. Even in the outside world he has to function as a centre, as a channel of the Divine Being. It is not for him to seek any lesser destiny. Sri Aurobindo observes in a classic sentence that to conquer the lures of egoistic life on earth is the first victory. To conquer the lure of individual happiness in a heaven beyond is the second victory. The third and the final victory is to conquer the lure for escape from the stress and strife of cosmic life. Life has a meaning; the individual is given a consciousness, a scope and a field. To realise that meaning, help others to realise in their own lives the meaning, and manifest according to his capacity, in the mode of his nature is the Divine Intention. And ultimately, whatever destiny the individual chooses, it is related to the relation between his soul and Nature. The soul has to liberate itself; there are a hundred ways to effect that liberation, but it has to use that liberty, the freedom so gained, to conquer Nature, master Nature, to direct it to bring about the fulfillment of the Divine Will in the terrestrial universe.

Any questions?

Is there a spiritual significance to the fact that there are more people on the earth now than there ever have been before in the history of the earth?

It only testifies to the fact that this is a growing creation. Every moment new energies, new souls are being released into manifestation from the Divine Source. It is only a few who choose to cancel themselves and draw back into what they call Nirvana. But there is a continuous blossoming forth, an emergence of truth-ideas, truth-lines, truth-force, souls carrying the Divine Spark into manifestation.

If today you find many, tomorrow you are going to find many more. All the artificial methods of limiting the number are not going to make much differnce for the simple reason that the number of souls that this Mother Earth can sustain is much more than we can conceive. It is because the resources of earth have not been properly tapped and exploited that there is this imbalance and the loud lament of overpopulation. Till the optimum number that the earth can support is reached, this process will continue. In a sense, it is illusory to speak even of this optimum number, for as the consciousness spreads, even the capacity of the earth will increase. Once the Mother pointed out that as the supramental force organises itself and digs into matter, the whole plant world will turn greener. There will be more life-force, more lasting and more powerful. So the earth will become more productive as Divinity enters it and unveils itself progressively.

Every moment new souls are entering into the "race to God" to quote from *Savitri*.

In Savitri, in the section that preceeds the arrival of "the omnipotent flaming pioneer", comes the giant dance of Shiva clearing the path. Now is this a prophecy of the destruction that will preceed the new creation? We hear from those who have gone to America, for example, of the state of deep depression in which it is psychologically, of the increase of violence, the hold ups of gangsters, the glorifying of them in films and so forth, and some Aurovillians have written back that there is a feeling of insanity. Does the increase of souls in subjection, as it were, in slavery, indicate that there will be this giant dance of Shiva?

The giant dance is over; the destruction is over already. The whole of the old civilisation has been destroyed. Psychologically, physically, the old civilisation is dead. The two wars, and the revolutions in the minds of men have destroyed all the old values. It is the radiant new creation that is to form itself; the present is an interim period and what we see are only surface phenomena of the transitional period when the old is gone and the new has not yet come.

In the larger perspective, after all, what are these little violences, little disturbances? Why don't you see the positive aspect of the whole thing? All over the globe, the Truth-Force is at work bringing out all falsehood, exposing it to ridicule, forcing men to search their hearts, forcing them to give up sham, to turn a new leaf in their lives, convincing people of the absurdity of their old ways.

There is, presiding over each individual evolution, what in Sri Aurobindo's philosophy is called the central being. In Indian terms it is called the Jivatman; for our purpose Sri Aurobindo's characterisation of it as the central being is enough. Now, this central being is always above the evolution; it stands above supporting it, witnessing it. It is, however, not altogether above because it projects a small emanation of itself into this evolution. That central being is always in touch with the parent Divine. There are millions of central beings, all of them are derived directly from the manifesting Divine and are in touch, linked with it. Now each central being projects a ray of itself, an emanation of itself in this movement of individual evolution. This emanation is called the psychic. It is a point of consciousness linked to the central being and therefore linked with the Divine Consciousness. Gradually, by evolution, by the gathering of experience, this essence becomes an entity. This entity life after life, further develops into what is called a being, the psychic being.

Now, this psychic being may be loosely called the soul. There is a part of the soul which is the Self, standing behind. There is a part which is involved and growing in evolution. Now that part of the soul which is involved in evolution and growing in evolution is called the psychic being. So for our purpose we may say that the soul which is involved in evolution is the psychic being; the soul that is not involved, but stands behind is what the Upanishads call the Self. It is not involved, but it has to support that which is involved. So there are three: there is the central being, Jivatman; there is the Self, the Atman; there is the psychic being which is the psychic purusha or the soul involved in evolution.

This psychic being grows by experience and as it grows in consciousness it develops many personalities. The more it develops, the more the personalities it gathers, it grows nearer the Divine. The climax in its evolution is reached when, in the process of growth and expansion, the psychic being links with the Jivatman, with the central being. In a sense, that is the end of individual Sadhana. Thereafter, whatever is to evolve is left entirely to the Divine Will. But until that happens there is the necessity for personal effort, personal aspiration. Until the individual's psychic being links up with the divine portion above, he has to make the effort. Thereafter the Divine takes charge.

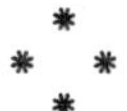

Instrumental personality: personality is mental personality, vital personality, physical — all these. The psychic being expresses itself, builds, so to say, these personalities — it stands behind and the more personalities it is able to organise around itself, the more evolved, the more mature it becomes. It may not carry to the next birth a personality it builds in this life, but the essence of the experience of these personalities forms part of its capital for the next birth.

* * * *

The Jivatman is above. The Atman is a projection of the Jivatman, standing behind. It is not above. The Self of an individual, what is called the Atman, is behind, it is not above. Above, behind, in front, you may say there are so many poises, necessary in the course of manifestation. It is a way of putting things. The central being, the Jivatman, standing behind, is the Self, Atman. It is an emanation. But again, we are using human language to describe a superhuman phenomenon. There can be no part, but for the sake of clarification, for our understanding in terms of the intellect, we have to say it is a portion; just as we say the central being is a portion of the Divine, the psychic being, the soul is an emanation of the central being.

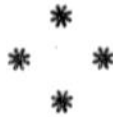

When you become conscious of the Self, you feel separate from all movement, from all Nature. You are alone, passive, in peace — undisturbable peace — nothing else exists at that time. When you experience the central being, you get a sense of freedom coupled with the action of overseeing, for it oversees all that goes on. Along with freedom, there is a vertical dimension to the experience of the central being. When you become conscious of the Self, you automatically become conscious of the Self of others, because the Self is extended everywhere, the same Self everywhere. So at that level you experience a sort of horizontal unity with the whole universe. In the psychic being, when you experience it, there is emphasis on the individual aspect of manifestation.

Still some doubt? I think if you read the section on the psychic being, the central being, in the *Letters* by Sri Aurobindo — the first volume — things will be clearer after what we have discussed, Sri Aurobindo has developed the philosophy of the psychic more in letters than he has in *The Life Divine* or the *Synthesis*. The practical aspect of it is in the *Letters*. In *The Life Divine*, I think he has emphasised that it is a projection of the Bliss-Self. There are, you know, five selves — the physical Self, the vital Self, the mental Self, the Knowledge Self, the Bliss Self. There are so many what we call 'bodies' in man, each ensouled by the particular Self. At the inmost depth, there is what is called the Bliss-Self and the psychic being is the deputy of the Bliss-Self.

You might look up "The Double Soul in Man" in *The Life Divine*, first volume. But first read well the section on the psychic being in the *Letters*. He has been extremely categorical in his definitions there, because this concept of the psychic being and its philosophy is not there in Indian philosophy nor in Western philosophy. What is called the "psyche" in Greek thought is quite different from what Sri Aurobindo means.

You spoke of the many ways of liberation of the soul. Where does he indicate this?

The yogic tradition is there, the mystic tradition is there. There are traditional ways of liberating oneself through the way of knowledge, through the way of love, through the way of works, through the way of the pursuit of sound, through the way of a progressive dissolution of the nature part of oneself, dispossessing oneself of all that is not properly disposed so that only the soul remains. It remains until that too is joyously dissolved in the vaster soul of Existence. There is Mother's and Sri Aurobindo's way which combines the principles of most of these paths so that any individual can start where it is natural for him, and derive support and help from all the personalities of his being and formulations of his nature. In a sense Sri Aurobindo's yoga is the easiest, just as in another sense it is the most difficult. It is easy because one doesn't rely upon one's own effort; one has only to be sincere, and open oneself to the higher yogic power, the Divine Power to work on one's being. That does the sadhana; the human effort is a supporting action, a sustaining activity. All that is required is sincerity and surrender. But it is difficult because one is called upon to change one's nature. This change of nature is essentially a personal effort. Here the Divine can sustain, can guide, can help, but he cannot effect the change itself. The human will has to do it. There comes the most difficult part of Sri Aurobindo's yoga, and both the processes are so interwoven that after a certain stage is reached, the next door cannot be opened to the descent of the still higher force unless some change is made in our nature. So it is a combined endeavour of the human and the Divine.

We could say that the central being presiding over the evolution of each individual is an individual poise of the Divine. So each Jivatman is conscious not only of its unity with the parent Divine, but of its oneness with the several central beings on earth. When it projects itself, puts an emanation of itself in individual evolution necessarily that emanation has the character of the central being. There is a part that is conscious of its union with others, and a part that is involved for experience. That is the psychic being, that is the Self and overseeing both the formulations of itself is the central being.

The psychic being stands behind.

Behind, behind — it is our job to bring it out. The psychic being stands behind, the psychic world also stands behind the gradation of worlds. The psychic *world* is not on one of the many planes that each one has to ascend; it stands behind supporting all. It is the soul. In the individual context also the psychic stands behind supporting the physical, the vital, the mental; all the three form a nodus, as it were, in the psychic being. It should be the endeavour of every seeker to gradually open the way and draw out the psychic being to come to the front. By aspiration, by creating the necessary climate of Truth, Harmony, Love in our external being, an attempt is made to draw out a ray of the psychic being. It comes, strikes the outer surface, withdraws, appears again, and gradually the influence of the psychic percolates to the surface. By cultivation, by extension of the area on which this influence can act, the field is created for the psychic being itself to eventually emerge and assume the captaincy of the ship of life.

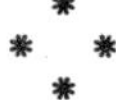

The inconscient does not enter into the scheme of the Tantras to which Sri Aurobindo makes mention in his writings. The ancients never went down to that level, they just described it metaphorically as the "world's underground". They speak of seven or fourteen worlds, one below the other, describe them as worlds of darkness, worlds of glittering wealth, worlds of enjoyment, worlds of perpetual misery, and so on. But they never brought it into the scheme of transformation. They spoke of change only on the levels above the subconscient. So these are two different contexts. The question of the inconscient arrives only when transformation of the kind Sri Aurobindo and Mother envisage is effected. It is a wholesale transformation, transmutation, of human nature into a Divine nature. This was not admitted quite as a practical possibility in the ancient systems. They admitted it as a theoretical possibility, but all agreed ultimately, that the physical is a stumbling block and there is nothing to be done with it. There are sciences in India — there were at any rate — which attempted by combining yoga and medicine, particularly using certain compounds of mercury, herbal juices and the like, to change the physical substance of the body into something that would transcend death. It was only an attempt, mechanical means were used to reach an end that is above mechanism, that is why it did not succeed.

16

Planes of our Existence

We were speaking of the relations between soul and Nature, between Purusha and Prakriti, as they are termed in Indian philosophy. We also saw that the soul has to acquire full domination over Nature. That is possible only by the soul uniting with the Divine Purusha, the Divine Soul in the universe, and it is only by this identity arrived at between the individual purusha and the Divine that it is possible to bring Nature under complete control.

But as we function on earth, the reverse is the case. The soul is completely subject to nature; even when we think we have mastery over nature, it is only a subtle slavery. The freedom, the domination is more mental than real. Even on the mental plane, there is a mental nature to which the mental soul is subject. How then are we to achieve this full liberation of soul and the subsequent mastery of the soul over Nature? Certainly it is not possible on earth as it is constituted. It can only be possible, logically, in some other world, where the soul is not so hopelessly subject to nature, where things are more flexible and free; or there must be in our own being, in our own consciousness, levels of existence — called planes of consciousness — where it is possible to establish different relations with Nature.

In the traditional yoga of knowledge the reason stands between the earth-world, the world in which we live — where the soul is completely lost in Nature — and the spiritual plane of existence, the spiritual world where the soul is not subject. May be it is not the master, but it is not subject to Nature. Once the reason makes this demarcation, the spiritual will, the central will steps in and detaches the being from involvement in Nature in the world and sets the soul free. No doubt in the course of this transition the soul perceives that there are many other levels of existence that it has not negotiated simply because they are irrelevant to its purpose. Certain traditions even state that they are not only irrelevant but dangerous because the experiences that these planes of existence yield to the soul are distracting, illusive, disruptive and the straight-eyed soul prefers to ignore them. But this narrow path is not open to the seeker of the integral path. Even as God accepts the whole universe with its several planes, and the several worlds of each plane, he who seeks to realise God in his totality has got to accept, has got to embrace the universe in all its totality. This province of knowledge of the various planes of existence, the gradations of the cosmic being, is properly called the field of occult science. In the West it was cultivated in detail, whereas in the East it never formed a separate subject by itself for the simple reason that, for the Eastern mind, nothing was truly occult. Each one was interrelated with the other spheres of existence, and one had only to turn the attention to which ever side one chose in order to know it better.

All the same, these planes of existence have been given different systems of classification in the different traditions of the world. According to the approach, according to the goal, according to the process that is chosen, certain aspects of this occult knowledge are emphasised in one system, passed over in another. Sri Aurobindo chooses the system that has been handed down by the seers of the Veda and, if we may say so, explicitly stated in the great line of the Upanishads. He prefers this because this system of classification has been done with a view to help our objective of liberation — liberation from ignorance, liberation from involvement in the lower nature. According to this system, the whole manifestation is conceived as being based on seven principles, seven principles of existence beginning from our end with the body, the life and the mind — based upon the principles of matter, life-force and mind. Above there are the eternal, uncreated worlds or planes of Existence, Consciousness and Bliss, Saccidananda. Linking them is the plane of Truth-Consciousness, called the Supermind. These seven principles are interwoven, they are not separate from each other really, but they are so many demarcated principles of manifestation. You would ask, as it has been asked so often: What exactly is a plane of existence? What do you mean by plane of consciousness? A "plane," in this context, means a particular poise of the soul related to its nature. The poise taken by the soul and the relations that are built up between nature and soul differ from level to level of existence. So where a particular type of relation obtains, where there is one fixed poise of relation between the soul and nature, that is recognised as a plane of existence. On each plane there can be many worlds; it will not do to confuse a plane and a world. A plane of consciousness is a vast expanse of existence where there may be different worlds with different stresses, but based fundamentally on the same principle that governs that plane of existence.

Existence, Sri Aurobindo points out, always contains three terms implicit in it on whatever plane you approach it.. There is first the sheer existence; what exists is conscious on its own, at its core it is conscious. Whether on the surface the consciousness is manifest or not, articulate or not, within the existence there is the awareness. This awareness, further, is not a static awareness. It is a forceful awareness; the awareness extends itself as a force, as a power, and this power or force functions to affirm the delight of existence. Existence is there, self-aware, spreading itself in force for a purpose. That purpose is to express and to affirm its delight of existence on the plane on which it is organised. So whatever the plane of existence, these three terms — Existence, Consciousness and Bliss or Delight — are present, latent or patent. This plane of earth, the physical earth on which we live is the first plane with which we are concerned. Here the poise of soul-and-nature is fixed; the soul is completely involved in nature, consciousness is completely involved in a poise which appears to be one of inconscience, delight is buried in insentience. So the characteristic feature of our plane of existence, of the earth on which we live is one of complete involution, complete subjection to nature.

The purpose of life there is to evolve what is involved, to unveil what is hidden. The whole struggle for existence, as it is called, is towards this end, to release the soul from its entire subjection to nature, to awake consciousness from its sleep, to free the impulse of delight from the swoon of insensibility in which it is imprisoned. This is the character of the material plane based upon matter, on which our world on earth is organised. If this were all, there would be no hope of liberation for the soul on earth. If this were the entire pattern, the entire framework, man could never hope to get liberation. But this plane of existence, the material plane, is not alone as we have seen. It is only one plane, one gradation of a large system in which there are other gradations overtopping the material.

Above the material, there is another plane differently organised, with a different poise of the soul, as regards to nature. This is governed by the life principle. If inertia, stability is the feature of the material plane, movement, flexibility is the feature of the life plane. If, on earth, it is the form that is more important, that determines the action of the life-energy of the consciousness, on the life plane it is the life-force, the life-energy that determines what form it will have. Existence is freer, forms change, there is a more rapid movement, there is a greater release and more adaptability in the relation of the soul with nature. The soul, when it takes its poise on the life plane, is called the vital purusha, the vital soul.

This plane is definitely and infinitely larger than the material plane. We are apt to think that the earth is boundless, because the physical universe is so vast, but the subtler vital plane is vaster; it envelops the physical, is much larger, has more freedom, and it has its subplanes. There are those nearer this material earth — almost melting into the subtle earth, subtle physical, even as there are those above which touch the mental plane. The experience of the soul is correspondingly different from subplane to subplane. On the subplane touching the physical are the intensities of the heavens and the hells constructed by human imagination. It is a superstition that heaven and hell are permanent locations somewhere in existence. Actually they are our own projections — projections of our own thoughts, imaginations, desires and passions on the vital plane, on the life plane — where they form on the strength of our projection. If we withdraw our support, they just dissolve. Each person creates his own heaven and his own hell; they are not cosmic provinces — a heaven where the virtuous go and a hell where the sinners are thrown. They are individual formations which thrive in the vital world. Similarly, in the higher worlds of the vital plane, there are the mental heavens, the psychic heavens, the ideal worlds, a reflection of the ideal world which the pure mind imagines, constructs in its dealing in ideas. So the vital plane is a variegated part of the universe where there is more freedom, but still the soul continues to be subject to the vital nature.

As we said, each plane has its own projection of the soul and of nature. Both share in the characteristic of the plane on which they are functioning. The physical earth, the physical world, is in a sense a projection of certain movements on the vital plane. When vital movements seek to realise themselves in conditions other than their own, it is the material world that gets erected. To put it more philosophically, it is as a result of pressure from the life-world that life forms itself in this material world, and manifests there.

In each person there is the projection of the vital world, the life world. What we are conscious of as the desire-self — our personality that seeks to acquire, to enjoy, to dominate, to aggrandise — is only the surface projection of the life-self within us. The larger part of the life-self is behind; it is called in Sri Aurobindo's philosophy the true and the inner vital being.

Just as this life-world and life-plane has its own basis of manifestation, there is above it the mental plane where mind is the ruler, not life-force but mentality. The mental consciousness determines all movements — not only in its own world but through the life-force below it influences and forms itself in the physical worlds as the physical mind. In this realm of the mental plane, the movement is still faster, more free. Time and space are not so binding as in the physical world. When the mental principle or the mental soul projects itself in the vital world it takes on the character of desire and becomes the desire mind or the vital mind on the vital plane, and when it reaches in the course of its manifestation the material world, it becomes the physical mind. As with the vital being on the mental plane also there is the surface mentality, the surface mind which is somewhat superficial and behind it is a larger mind which functions somewhat differently. It is not restless in its thinking activity; it is calm, still, and for the greater part it reflects what comes from above.

Far above the mind there are still other planes of existence — what are called the spiritual planes or the occult hemisphere. We are not conscious of them because they are not yet organised, in the evolutionary sense, in our being.

The Upanishads speak of the physical sheath, the vital sheath, the mental sheath, and thereafter the knowledge sheath and the bliss sheath. This knowledge sheath and the bliss sheath are really two aspects of the causal body — what we may call in Sri Aurobindo's terminology the supramental body — which is not yet organised in the human system. Still, some influence from that plane touches man indirectly. Till recently it used to be indirect, through the various intervening planes of existence between mind and supermind. It is only now, at this hour in evolution, that a ray of the supramental light is able to act directly in the mind, and when the physical mind receives the supramental light directly it is called the mind of light. The mind of light is already formed; it is functioning. Whoever reaches that stage of evolution can embody it. But the supramental light has not yet become part of the physical existence in the sense in which it can be a permanent acquisition for anyone who strives. For that, in principle, the material transformation has to be achieved.

From Questions and Answers

In the present discussion we have been concerned only with these three planes of existence, because it is on these planes that we still live, and on which we have to work out the freedom of the soul from nature and acquire, on these levels, a certain mastery so that nature becomes a vehicle of the soul.

Those worlds refer to the upper hemisphere, Sat, Chit, Ananda. It is those three that project themselves and create themselves in different conditions as the worlds of matter, worlds of life, and worlds of mind. In that sense the lower three worlds are created worlds — created in the course of evolutionary process. But the worlds of Sat, Chit, Ananda are there irrespective of whether the evolutionary movement is there or not. They are called in Indian philosophy the Eternal Uncreate. We call them worlds in our terms: actually they are the presentation of the Supreme Reality about which we can know nothing. When It lends Itself to be perceived and experienced by the human consciousness, we see them as the eternal worlds, as the eternal aspects of the Reality, as Saccidananda. We call them worlds, but they are not really worlds in our sense.

But are they worlds where there is a permanent existence?

They are. They are permanent worlds, because actually it is one organisation, one system presenting three aspects. It is a triple world. That is why some systems don't speak of seven planes of existence, seven worlds, but of five worlds — the lower three, the supramental and then in one block Saccidananda. They don't distinguish the latter as three, and for spiritual experience that is more true. It is for the understanding of our logical intelligence that we speak of seven worlds, but actually, in spiritual realisation, after the supramental, it is all bliss.

Even though it's all bliss, is that the area that Sri Aurobindo experienced where he saw not the Timeless but the endless Time in the permanent sense of existence?

This Bliss principle, this Ananda is manifest on each plane of existence. When you touch a certain depth, whether in matter, or in life-force or in the mind, you experience that delight principle — uncaused delight throbbing, flowing on its own without any cause. So each seer, each saint, each realised man, when he seeks the delight, gets it on the plane of his realisation. The Advaitic experience that Sri Aurobindo had was on that altitude of being where the mind falls utterly silent, and there is a possession by the Impersonal. There there is the permanent peace and the ineffable bliss. Go still higher and there will be a bliss and a delight appropriate to that plane. That is why the Mother says in one of her prayers in the *Prayers and Meditations* that we have to construct a harmony of the various delights on the various levels of our being.

Then there's no permanent existence on those planes?

These three are there on every plane in principle — Existence, Consciousness, Bliss.

But they're not permanent constructions.

They're self-existent. They are permanent there, but even here they project themselves, try to formulate themselves in different conditions.

There's no projection on their own plane.

There is no projection, it is only a self-existence. There they are self-existent, here they have to manifest. You can't realise on the material plane the Saccidananda that is self-existent. You can only realise it as it manifests on earth.

These have to have a prototype, don't they?

The prototype is there.

Yes, but they have to have their self in its own state, self-realised and constructed, don't they?

They construct themselves here in different patterns. The world of existence, the principle of existence there which is uncreated throws itself here in different conditions and creates the material world.

I see; when you said the uncreated worlds, I thought you meant that they were worlds that had never been created but had always existed.

The worlds of the upper hemisphere are not created by any creative Godhead. They are antecedent to evolution. In whatever cycle — the present cycle is a cycle of evolution, but you have to conceive of other cycles where the principle may not be one of evolution — those worlds of Existence, Consciousness and Bliss are always there because they are the Absolute as turned towards manifestation. They are eternally existent in themselves; they do not need to enter into the movement of manifestation. Here in our world, they have to pass through the process of evolution to be perfect. There they are eternally perfect.

Then there's no construction.

There there is no construction; here there is construction.

Then that's the Unmanifest that we are talking about.

In the Unmanifest there are not even worlds. You can't even say there is Existence-Consciousness-Bliss. When what is unmanifest turns towards manifestation, the first experience you have is of this triple Saccidananda.

To reach the level of the causal body, because of Sri Aurobindo's pioneering for us, all we need to do is the aspiring and surrendering to receive it, the calling and the receptivity?

Yes, formerly even if people had done all this, they couldn't have realised the Supramental. But now that the passage is laid, and it has been linked with the earth-consciousness, it is a possibility open to all to try for. Till now it was a concept.

Are you aware of any positive effects of Mother's withdrawal on the acceleration of inner development recently?

Yes, the inner contact is more easy. There is a continuous contact, no gap, and things get done almost with the same facility as was possible when physical contact with her was available. There is less agitation in the atmosphere, more calm — which is inexplicable to outsiders — and an increase of faith.

Where will the physical body go?

Why should the physical body go? The physical body has to change. Where did Mother's mind go? The content of the mind is different, so the content of this body will be different. The outer frame may be there, but the content will be different.

How did the mind of light then operate in the Mother?

It has been operating for the last so many years. The action of the supramental light in the physical mind is the mind of light.

Physical mind?

Physical mind; there are three gradations, the pure mind, the vital mind and the physical mind, aren't there? Broadly, these are the three levels of the mind — let us leave the subdivisions — mind proper, mind in the vital, mind in the physical.

This action of light then is the actual beginning of the transformation of the cells in her body?

You can say so. When the mind of light gets formed, that is the beginning of the actual transformation of the physical. You start from the physical mind level.

In contacting Mother inwardly, in coming into relation with her does the content of our consciousness affect her or is she protected against our incursions this way?

There is a self-protecting mechanism which makes her aware of the quality of the consciousness that contacts her. But the things fall back.

So our answer comes in relation to the quality of our own consciousness?

Whatever the quality of our consciousness, as long as the approach is sincere, the Grace responds.

17

The Lower Triple Purusha

We completed our discussion of the series of worlds in the cosmos and the series of planes in the being of man when we met last. We saw that these series are like a ladder of planes with the worlds upon them plunging deep into Matter, and perhaps even deeper, and rising to the highest heights of cosmic existence and projecting even higher into some supracosmic Absolute as some philosophies avow.

Man is not normally aware of these several planes of existence in himself or in the world for the simple reason that his whole life is based upon, organised and governed by his material consciousness. His life is based upon matter, and it is within the organisation of matter that he functions. Looked at from this point of view, man appears to be like an insignificant speck in the huge totality of the physical universe. There is indeed a great and mighty movement of time in which his own life looks like an insignificant hour. Wherever he looks around, he sees a mask of forms, movements, thrown pell-mell, getting shaped into some sort of order by the working of certain self-existent laws which he does not at first understand. He tries to understand these laws of the physical universe in order, first, that he may tune himself to them, and, second, that by understanding them, he can better govern his life and eke out some sort of pleasure in his life-time. This picture reduces human life either to a phenomenon of automatism or something at the mercy of external forces. Physical science gives him certain understanding of the external laws of the universe and some sort of grasp of the functioning of his surface mind and vitality, but little more. However, man has glimpses, undeniable glimpses, in himself of another order of existence beyond the physical. He feels those moments, he intuits them, though he cannot explain them In some gifted individuals these perceptions of the orders of existence that are beyond the physical take a definite shape and govern their life-movement. Just as the laws of physical science explain physical phenomena, these individuals seek to understand and to explain to themselves the various occult phenomena into which they are given glimpses.

That is why whenever there is an efflorescence of material prosperity and civilisation, a full cultivation of the physical sciences, that period is invariably followed by one in which human interest is in occult science, in matters pertaining to supraphysical reality. And religion is one such quest.

Religions affirm the existence of the supraphysical worlds, supraphysical beings as related to man. They confirm and strengthen his perception of other movements, other beings than the physical. Religions also show the way to bridge the gulf between the physical and the supraphysical. They assure for man a better and a happier life in the beyond; the present existence is not all, it can be followed by a larger and a greater existence. Some religions, however, deny any past to the present life. They do not admit any kind of past immortality to the being, but assure man that if he takes a particular path, accepts a particular dogma, he has a chance of living in an immortal existence hereafter. There are other religions which do not take so narrow a view, but accept a past and a future to the present. They conceive of the being of man as a developing soul which evolves, step by step, Godward and pursues a line of development which culminates in a totally different order of life than the one that is open to man at present.

Some philosophies have it that the Divinity, the Godhead, is something eternally separate from the evolving soul, and the highest that the soul can conceive for itself is to adore the Divine, live in proximity to the Divine, serve the Divine, but never unite with the Divine. There are, on the other hand, other philosophies, other religions which say that the Divine can be united with, that the soul itself is a spark of the Divinity. As it grows, it can attain identity with its parent Flame. There are still others which speak of the Divine as something impersonal, an impersonal Absolute in which one can only merge. Once you merge there is no further individuality — that means once you depart from the life on earth you have no further life.

Sri Aurobindo accepts the vision and the perception that the Divine is all of these. The Divine is not imprisoned in the personal status, or the impersonal aspect. It is both and transcends either. It is open to man, it is open to the human soul to choose its line of union with the Divine. It can choose to play at being separate in the background of unity. It can, in one part of itself, repose in the Impersonal, in the eternal status, participating at the same time in the dynamic personality of the Divine.

In this total view, the Divine is approached not only to be united with somewhere else, but to be embraced in its relations with the universe which it has put forth from itself.

With this background, when we study the different gradations of the individual and the cosmic existence, the first fact we see inescapably is the materiality of life. The purusha and the prakriti, the soul and nature, are at play in the material field. Whatever consciousness has evolved there, it is always occupied with material interests. It never goes beyond the material horizon. In the human being there is a touch of mentality, there is a surface play of vitality but both mind and life are subservient to the physical.

In his normal existence man is essentially a physical purusha, a physical soul with certain mental and vital energies serving that physical. And as long as man continues to live in this state that is predominantly physical, when he dies he cannot go beyond the series of physical planes. He cannot gain access to the planes of higher vital worlds or mental worlds. The soul that is essentially physical, that is constantly encased in the physical, cannot go beyond the last ranges of the physical world, the subtle physical. Thereafter it has to come back to the physical earth, work out possibilities, develop its finer side, develop its vital and mental content before it is in a position to go higher in its transition after death.

If care is taken to bring about a promotion of the vital and the mental content in the personality of man, then he becomes aware that the physical purusha is not all. There is, beyond the physical self, a larger self, the self of the life-force — what is called in the Indian philosophy the self of prana. There is a vivid description in one of the Upanishads — the Taittiriya Upanishad — of these several selves in the being of man. Here is a description of the physical self, which we have just discussed. (In the Upanishadic thought, food denotes matter.)

> Verily, all sorts and races of creatures that have their refuge upon earth are begotten from food. Thereafter they live also by food, and it is to food again that they return at the end at last. For food is the eldest of created things, and therefore they name it the Green Stuff of the Universe.
>
> Verily, they who worship the Eternal as food attain the mastery of food to the uttermost. Food is the eldest of created beings, and therefore they name it the Green Stuff of the Universe. From food all creatures were born, and being born they grow by food. Lo, it is eaten and it eats; it devours the creatures that feed upon it. Therefore it is called food from the eating.
>
> Now behind this Self of food, there is a second and inner

> Self which is other than this that is of the substance of food, and it is made of the vital stuff called prana. And the Self of prana fills the Self of food. Now the Self of prana is made in the image of man, according as is the human image of the other, so is it in the image of man. The gods live and breathe under the dominion of prana and men and all these that are beasts, for prana is the life of created things and therefore they name it the life-stuff of the All.
>
> Verily, they who worship the Eternal as Life, reach life to the uttermost, for prana is the life of created things and therefore they name it the life-stuff of all. And this Self of prana is the soul in the body of the former one which was of food.

Deeper than the physical Self, is the vital Self. This vital Self — of which we are not yet fully aware but of which we are aware only indirectly through its projection in the form of desires, movements of life-force — is organised on its own plane, the life plane. Just as the physical purusha is organised on the physical plane whereupon we live, the vital Self is fully organised on its own plane. But it does not get the scope and the facility to function on its own in man as long as he stations himself on the level and the base of the physical.

In the measure in which, by his inner discipline, by some means, he separates himself from his physical involvement, separates and rises above the physical Self, he becomes conscious of the vital Self. He finds himself in the vortex of a mighty movement of life-force and energies which fill the universe. He has the feeling of something in him floating in the universe, alone with the life-force. He becomes aware and he perceives how the different subtle energies behind the physical are at work in this world. By his will he can direct his part of the vital energies on others. He who has acquired a certain individuality in the vital realm, who has contacted the source of vital energies in his own soul, can direct the healing forces of vitality towards those who are in need of it. Those who are sick, those who are mentally sick, those who need to feel the joy of life — all those can be influenced, they can be helped by one who has access to this vital purusha. In other words, one who activises his vital purusha in his living personality, who dynamises the vital force in his nature, towards him others turn. Because when they come within his ambience they feel uplifted in a certain way, they feel nourished. But that is not all.

Going deeper, one realises that this vital energy itself is directed by another purusha, another soul, another Self, the mental Self. As the same Upanishad observes:

> Now, there is yet a second and inner Self, which is other than this that is of prana, and it is made of mind. And the Self of mind fills the Self of prana. The Self of mind is made in the image of man . . .The delight of the Eternal from which words turn away without attaining, and the mind also returns baffled, who knows the delight of the Eternal? And this Self of mind that knows the delight is the soul in the body to the former one which was of prana.

This mental Self is beyond the range of most, because it is the mental Self which projects itself into the vital world and, secondarily into the physical. In the mind, one comes very much nearer the Reality of Existence. Not the physical mind, of course, but in the core of the stuff of mind there is the Self. This mental purusha, as it is called in Indian philosophy, when given scope to organise itself in one's existence, uplifts the physical Self, enlightens the vital Self. There is a stream of Light, a stream of harmony proceeding from the mental Self. When one is aware of the action of the mental Self, one perceives a large realm of ideas and thoughts looming over the physical universe. An infinite number of possibilities that are released in the universe are seen. The division that is so inconvenient on the physical plane is absent on the mental plane. In the measure in which the mental purusha is real to me, my mind reflects what goes on in your mind, and wherever I will it, my mind grasps what is in the particular mind that I want to know. There is a continuous interchange which can be made conscious. One can influence the thoughts of others, project one's own thoughts into other minds with greater facility. This is the awakening and the activising of the mental purusha.

These three — the physical Self, the vital Self and the mental Self — which are organised and can be made active in man with yogic effort, constitute the lower triple Self. Even after all these three are cultivated, man is still in the realm of the triple world of ignorance. The shadow of ignorance is still there because nature, prakriti, still rules the purusha. The Self has not obtained a mastery over the nature as long as it is confined to this triple formula of matter, life and mind. The soul has to exceed this formula, get beyond it in order to get real liberation and victory over nature leading to an eventual transformation of nature.

That will be the theme of our next talk.

Any questions?

In regard to the intermediate state – after death and before the next birth – what is the development needed in order to attain the higher altitudes of that intermediate stage?

The after-death state entirely depends upon the state of consciousness that is developing during life on earth. If our vision, our interests, our consciousness are entirely physical, with the life and the mind only as an annex to the physical, the soul cannot go beyond the frontiers of the subtle-physical. If it develops here a mental life, becomes conscious of the vital life, directs it, makes the vital and the mental life real to itself, organises them, as Sri Aurobindo would say, around the self, governs them from the self, or in our language, builds up a vital and a mental personality, then alone can he get access to the vital and the mental worlds. As one develops and organises here on earth, one gets the passport, so to say, to enter those worlds above. Otherwise the soul fails to rise. It becomes too much for it. Just as an animal, when it dies, simply cannot go beyond the earth-atmosphere. It goes almost immediately back into another animal body. But once having arrived at the human stage, the soul automatically leaves the earth atmosphere and goes to the subtle physical; a further passage depends upon the consciousness that is developed here. If one has a certain mental life, a vital life and a little bit of soul life, say some devotion to God, belief in higher values, faith in beauty, love and such things that pertain to God, then he does get entry into those higher worlds which lead to the psychic.

It is said in certain scriptures that only by remembering God or repeating the name of God at the time of death can one go to the kingdom of God. But that is clearly an exaggeration. In the first place, one cannot be conscious of God at the moment of departure unless there has been during the life a background of God. A normal creature is either obsessed with fear of what happens after death or is rendered unconscious by the shock of death. It is only one who has lived some sort of spiritual life, has built up some spiritual past who can get into the spiritual poise at the time of leaving the body and thus ensure a smooth transition to the higher worlds, leading to the worlds of the spirit.

In Christianity there's the idea of last rites, where even if one has not been baptized into the Christian religion, he can be baptized just before death and be "saved". Could you comment on this?

As long as this sort of thing is only a religious ceremony, it has no spiritual significance. But if there is even a moment of repentance on the part of the person dying that is enough to ensure a departure from the past and to evoke a protecting influence from the guardian spirits. But this is irrespective of the religious ceremony; religious ceremonies have really no meaning in this context except when they have an effect of awakening in the dying person repentance and an asking for forgiveness from God. Normally they are treated as functions of the priest and are merely dry rituals.

You said that perhaps the most common state would be either unconsciousness or fear. Might it not also happen that a person has an opening in another direction?

What happens when such openings come is that the soul pushes forward. The soul within which is always conscious of the supra-physical realities, of the positive life beyond, casts a ray, a reflection and the mind opens to it. All this, provided, a man is in a condition to be conscious at that time. It is only a yogi or a person who is capable of certain detachment that can leave the body consciously. It is very rarely that people consciously depart from the physical body. They just lose consciousness and wake up after some time and do not even realise that they are dead. Many look for the body; and that is a time of great pain and confusions when they find that the body is not there. And all kinds of beings and elemental forces rush upon the defenceless soul. The subtle-physical body is defenceless. It is then if the habit has been made during the lifetime of remembering the Divine or the one who represents the Divine, that memory stands good stead. The call to the Divine is spontaneous and it acts as a light, as an armour, protecting the subtle-physical body from the multifarious attacks of the beings of the supra-physical worlds.

If one has dreamt beautiful dreams, emanated movements of love and harmony, thought well of everybody, one finds oneself in an ideal world where things are beautiful, harmonious. If on earth one has been accustomed all his life to find fault, criticise, to look always at the dark side of things, to surround himself always with dark thoughts, depressions, harmful imaginations — well he finds himself in what are called the sunless worlds.

These are the heavens and the hells of which religions speak and the traditions magnify. This is the sense in which Sri Aurobindo says that each man carries his own hell and heaven. As we sow here on earth, so we reap there. And each plane — the subtle physical the vital and the mental — has its own hells and heavens. If we are prisoners here of certain narrow ideas, narrow thoughts, if our thoughts are always poisonous, well, when we go to the mental world we will find ourselves in fetters from which we cannot break out until they are dissipated, until those meshes are broken; that is what is called working out the mental karma and shedding the mental sheath.

The shedding of each sheath is to neutralise and cancel the remnants of the karma that that particular part of the being acquired while on earth. They pursue one and it is only after all these sheaths are dissolved that one is free to go to the psychic world for rest.

You said something about the physical body having a form and the vital body having a form . . .

The physical *Self* having a form, the vital *Self* having a form, the mental *Self* having its own form.

What is the difference between mental Self and the mental body?

Self is what actuates the body.

Is that the soul?

At every level, the Supreme Self, individualised, poises itself as the Self and the Nature. On the physical, vital, mental, even on the spiritual levels, this double poising as nature and as soul is necessary for purposes of manifestation.

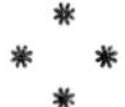

It is not everyone who can do it. Most who live in the physical have very little mental karma. How many really think? The mind that is active in a normal individual is the mental part of the physical, it is not the mind proper. The physical mind is active, the physical-vital, not the vital proper, not the mental proper. By yogic cultivation, by inner discipline, by separate compartmental organisation — as Mother describes — it is possible to develop these several personalities in man, the physical personality, the vital personality, the mental personality. They can be developed only by yoga; that is, the consciousness on each level is raised to its optimum. The individuality is developed, instead of remaining an inchoate mass.

Death is a negative conception and an integral yogin is always called upon to look to the positive side of everything. It is only as he dwells on the positive side that the negative loses its force, and once the yogin develops his life positively, death does not claim any thought, death reveals itself as but a process of life, a change of vesture. One thinks of death when one is afraid of death. In yoga there can be no fear of death because almost the first lesson is to separate oneself from nature and identify oneself with the soul which is immortal. So the more one becomes conscious of the immortal element in oneself, poises oneself in that consciousness, death loses its terror. Death can only provide an interesting field for research for those who are curious, but certainly it has no claim over the mind of man till all other subjects are exhausted. It is an area of darkness into which one need not enter until one is in possession of the supreme spiritual light, the Truth light, which lights up every little corner.

As a student of *Savitri*, you would have observed that the "The Book of Death" is hardly a few pages. It exposes death in its true colours; when death is brought too near the Light, death just dissolves.

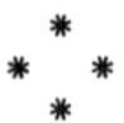

It was done not as a part of his individual yoga, but as a representative of the aspiring earth. Ashwapathy had to go through all the different levels of existence in order to have the experience and exhaust it and also so that he could have the right to call the Highest to come down. You must have seen that in his individual yoga, all these things are not mentioned. But when he starts as a traveller of the worlds on behalf of the collectivity, it is there that he is obliged to go down and down into the abysses of the sub-conscient, the inconscient till he touches the nadir of the depths. Only what is not described is what is beyond the nadir, the realms of light. It is Mother that has emphasised that aspect; I have not seen it in Sri Aurobindo's writings. She says it is global manifestation, so when you go down and down, just beyond there is the light. The light that is above, on the tops, that is here also. So when one emerges from those doors, one walks into the light.

18

The Ladder of Self-Transcendence

We ended last time on the subject of the lower triple purusha. We considered the three lower worlds with the three poises of Spirit presiding over them. We concluded that as long as we are in this triple formula, we continue to be under the shadow of ignorance. One has to exceed this lower triple formula and enter into the Transcendent. This is very much what the ancients call in the Veda breaking through the firmaments of heaven and earth, going beyond one's father and mother. For in the Veda, the heaven standing for the higher regions of the mind, is spoken of as the father and the material, the physical, is lauded as the mother. When the Veda speaks of breaking beyond the firmaments of heaven and earth, it means exceeding the lower triple existences and getting an entry into the higher triplicity of existence.

It is extremely difficult for the human mind to get a stable entry into the region beyond its highest summits. Even the lower levels of the higher existence — of which we are to speak later — is a feat for the mind if it can get lodging there. In the system of which we are speaking, the whole universe, the whole of manifestation, is divided into two halves, the upper half and the lower half, the lower consisting of the worlds of matter, life and mind, and the upper half consisting essentially of the worlds of sheer Existence, Consciousness-Force and Bliss, with the world of Truth-Light as the link between the two.

There in the higher hemisphere — the *parardha* as it is called, — is an illimitable manifestation of the glories of

Existence, the radiances of Consciousness and Force, the vast seas of Bliss. Here in the lower existence where we live normally, the Spirit is veiled, the glories of Existence, the brilliances of Consciousness, the floods of Bliss are veiled, kept in the background, and in the conditions of division, limitation and ignorance they are often expressed in almost contrary and even perverse forms like pain, suffering, limitation. It is essential for those who seek to cross into the freedom of the spirit to extend their being, step by step, to these higher realms of consciousness. And it is possible because these worlds that constitute the different spheres of existence are not independent separate entities but form — luckily for us — a gradation, a gradation of worlds on a series of planes.

As we observed in one of our talks, a plane is an organisation based on a particular principle of being. On that plane there can be any number of worlds, each stressing a certain aspect of that principle. So always a plane is a larger term than a world.

Now, Sri Aurobindo points out that on each plane, the Spirit or the manifesting soul takes a particular poise as regards its relation with Nature. Soul and Nature, the separable biune truth, take different poises in different principles of existence. To start from our end, when the Spirit or the being or the Soul, takes its poise in the principle of Matter, physical matter, we have what is called the material world. The material world is another name for a system of relations that develop between Soul and Nature when they are based on the principle of Matter. The very principle of matter is one of inertia, fragmentation, inconscience. Accordingly, the relations between the Soul and Nature on that plane are characterised by inertia, ignorance and division. From whichever direction you look at it, these characteristics of physical matter are inevitable in the relations between Soul and Nature based upon the physical principle.

In the universe the Spirit takes the material form. In the individual it becomes what is called the materialised soul, the soul that is encased in matter, that allows itself to be governed by the principle of Matter. This materialised soul, which is called in the Upanishads the *annamaya purusha*, has its own relations with the world. It dominates all the principles that are woven in the individual system. The life-force has to subserve to the needs of the physical; it limits itself to the frame that is provided for it by the material body. Similarly, the mind too is unable to function in its own right. It is constantly pulled down by the inertia and the ignorance that form the bedrock of material body. Neither the mind nor the life-force can function independently of the body as long as the dominant ruler in the life of man is the materialised soul. Even the spirit, the soul, that wants to manifest in this set of circumstances has to take account of the fragmentation and the inconscience that characterises this order of creation.

But the Spirit can poise itself also in the principle of Life as it has taken its base and organised itself in Matter. The Spirit organises itself in the matrix of the life-force. Movement, rapidity, self-effectuation, a certain amount of freedom, these are the characteristics of the life-force, the life-energy. And the Spirit that presides over this order of existence in the universe is the vital self, having relations with the vital nature.

Here also, in the individual context, the spirit becomes the vitalised soul, the *pranamaya purusha*. All its movements, all its perspectives are governed by the life-force in which it functions. Here it is the life-force that is the king; the body has to obey and respond to the pressures exerted upon it by the life-force. If the body cannot sustain the pressures, it breaks and the vital force chooses another vehicle. Similarly, even the mind, when it is connected with this vital soul, shares some of the fluidity that is a central feature of the vital self. Even the spirit gets more rhythm, gets more force of self-effectuation. But if one confines oneself to the level of the vital soul, vital nature, and does not seek to go beyond, it is desire, self-aggrandisement that come to rule. Man becomes, if not a slave of desire and life-energy, someone who uses life-energy ignorantly. He uses it for his own aggrandisement, for the fulfillment of his own desires. He is what is called in Indian terminology the *rakshasa* or the demon. A demon is a lower kind of titan. A titan, an *asura*, is he who can exercise any amount of self-control, do askesis, but for his own purpose, in order to gain dominion over others, to get himself on the throne. The asuric nature thrives on this misdirected world of life-energy.

Similarly, there is another plane where the Spirit can poise itself in its relations with Nature and that is the mental plane. Here the divisions, the limitations of physical matter, the material plane are not there nor the turbidities, the restlessness of the vital force; the mental levels, the levels of the mind, where the Spirit poises itself as the mental spirit or the mental self and mental nature, is nearer the original Spirit in man. That is why we say that to live in the mind is to live nearer the Spirit, for the mind is so constituted that under certain conditions it can reflect only the figure of Truth and not its body; still it is a great step in advance. The clarities of the higher mind, the sattwic luminosity that lights up the mental functioning, take one far ahead in the stair of evolution. Even then, both the life-force and the body find it a great strain to follow the quick steps of the mind. We are not speaking, at this moment, of the lower levels of the mind, the reasoning, logical, labouring, galley slave mind with which we are familiar, but the larger expanses and levels of mind touching the borders of the spiritual planes. These open up larger vistas, but still they are limitations. The mind cannot give us the final Truth. The mind can only be an instrument for the opening of the passage to the Truth. This is because it always divides, it always fragments, it always sees in bits, in strips and takes each strip for the whole, as Sri Aurobindo points out in *Savitri.*

The most that the pure mind can do is to impose its harmonies, however limited they may be, impose its clarities of light and understanding on the rest of the members of the being. Thereafter, the mind has to take a leap into the higher regions.

We have spoken of the materialised soul, the vital soul, the mental soul. We read last time from the Upanishads how besides the physical purusha there is another purusha and that is the life-soul. The life-soul, again encloses in itself the mind-soul, the mental purusha — but that's not the end. Behind the mental Self, forming the soul of the mental Self, there is called the knowledge Self. This knowledge Self is the poise of the Spirit on the principle of undeviating, unlimited knowledge. It is what is called *vijnana* in the Upanishads, what Sri Aurobindo calls the Real-Idea, the Supramental Consciousness, where Truth is plenarily manifest, where knowledge is self-evident and one doesn't have to labour for it. And knowledge is not separated from will; it carries in itself the power to effectuate what it sees and what it knows. This Power, the knowledge self, forms the knowledge sheath and, please note, this knowledge sheath which is finer, subtler and more complete than the mental sheath is the causal body. What is described as the causal body in Indian philosophy is this supramental sheath. In its deeper parts it turns into the bliss sheath. Knowledge-self on its summits reveals itself as bliss-self and this bliss-self is the foundation for the higher worlds, for the empire of the Saccidananda.

So the transition has to be effected from the mental to the knowledge self. That is precisely where the integral yoga comes in. All the traditional ways of yoga end with the leap of the human mind — the most developed mind — either into the transcendent silence of which the Buddha speaks, or into what appears as a non-existence in the infinite folds of the spirit to Shankara. It is a matter of controversy whether the mental soul that delivers itself in those regions continues its existence in any manner or it dissolves. The Mother has it that even when we say it is dissolved, in some way, it maintains its individuality. That is because this is the Will of the Supreme. When the Supreme emanated so many sparks out of himself, it was with a view to manifesting his glory in individual formations. When the individual soul returns it continues in principle, though not in form, in that stage where it is supposed to have dissolved itself. But this dissolution or immergence into silence, into non-existence, into Nirvana, into Bliss, is not the aim of the integral seeker. He has many more worlds to traverse. There are regions of consciousness and being that he has to reach, open himself to, receive into himself, organise in his being and manifest. As man is constituted at present, it is only the physical, the vital and the mental sheaths that are organised and functioning. The supramental or the causal sheath — the knowledge sheath — has to be built and added as a new dimension in man. This yoga is primarily meant to achieve this formation of the supramental body in man. Otherwise it remains a matter of mental knowledge. Unless it is made a constituent principle of our existence, a dynamic factor in our relations with our nature, with this world around, the knowledge sheath, the knowledge self cannot be said to have been operative in our life. In what way this knowledge-self is to be realised, made true and made a dynamic factor in our life, to what extent the past traditions hold the light and what is the contribution of Sri Aurobindo and Mother, will be our theme during the next talk.

You say that these souls merge themselves in silence, Nirvana – is this a permanent state, or is there any evolution past that?

In the systems that speak of the merger of the individual soul in those levels of consciousness, or Bliss, that is the end of evolution. What happens is the soul declines to traverse further on the ladder of evolution that is presented to it. It withdraws and retires, so to say, in complete peace or bliss. The contention of those philosophies is that it no more remains an individual, so there is no question of what it is going to do — it has no destiny, it has no evolution to carry out. Sri Aurobindo is the one thinker or seer who says that the final end of the soul is not to merge itself, to dissolve itself, but to retain its individuality and embody the divine consciousness. Mother says that even when you say it is dissolved, still the individual unit continues in principle in the being of the Supreme. Those systems like the Buddhist or the advaitic of Shankara don't believe in spiritual evolution, so for them the problem does not arise. They say the whole thing is a mistake. The Buddhists say there is no soul to evolve, it is all a bundle of impressions, desires, satisfactions, a sort of knot which we think is the soul, is the being. But there is no being, there is no soul. By a process of dissolution of desires, withdrawal from movements, all things are dissipated and the last knot of karma automatically dissolves and what is left is only Nirvana. Shankara says that as you dispossess yourself of this world and worldly impressions, as you withdraw from your involvement in the life-movement and get illumination by discrimination and study, by sadhana, the mind suddenly realises that all this is an illusion, a fantasy which is not real. The mind realises, "I am not bound, I am not dead, I am always free, I am the Eternal. There never was anything. If I thought there was, it was an imagination or a dream, a gigantic dream on the part of God". Even God is denied permanent validity in Shankara's philosophy. God, Ishwara, is a sort of president of this cosmos of Ignorance. So he also gets dissolved and only the Immutable, Absolute, Relationless, Ineffable Brahman remains and we attain our identity with Him. That is his philosophy.

How would you describe the role of the Matrimandir in this spiritual evolution?

Matrimandir, being a concrete expression of the Mother's consciousness and force, will always stand as a reservoir of inspiration, a lighthouse radiating continually the manifestation of Truth as is embodied in the Mother's body. What the Mother's embodiment is to us today will be the full-fledged Matrimandir to the whole of humanity. Does that make sense?

Yes. The chief architect of Auroville has said that it is his understanding from the Mother – and this fits in exactly with what you say – that the Matrimandir is to be the receptacle, the receiving station, of spiritual energy and of the Supramental Consciousness, that is, the Truth-Consciousness.

I would add: In the course of her life on earth, Mother has established links with so many levels of cosmic existence. Each of these links help those parts of the cosmic being to relate themselves to the Truth-Light. And this spiritual mechanism will also be embodied in the Mandir. What I mean to say is that it is not only the light and the consciousness that will be radiating from there but it will be providing the means also for each individual to realise them.

. . . *It's been very difficult for all as a whole and for each of us, is it that things will change hereafter?*

The crisis has come into the open in Auroville; it is slowly gathering elsewhere. All that I can say is that everything depends upon the will of the Supreme. Mother is not exerting herself either way. She has literally surrendered herself — her body, her mind, everything — to the Supreme. She refuses to make any movement on her own initiative. This is too profound and serious a moment for our minds to fathom. We have to wait. I don't know whether I said it here, but I once asked myself — not myself but Sri Aurobindo — in the early hours of the morning when I was on the sea beach, as to the why of this prolonged agony, physical agony of the Mother's. Why has she to go through it? The answer was quick: She continues because there is *still* a possibility. I understood;

that is her sacrifice. Then what is our duty, I asked. Throw your weight towards that possibility. Since then, personally I have no problem. He perceives that there is a possibility, he expects us to put our weight on the side of that possibility. Anyway, there is nothing that we little individuals can do in this matter. It is only the Supreme Will, as functioning in Sri Aurobindo for this purpose, that knows. The Mother does not know or she does not choose to know. Beyond this, I don't think I should say or can say anything.

In relation to this, more than a year ago there were a set of directives given by our Matrimandir workers to the Mother by Shyamsundar and signed with blessings by the Mother. This put a special responsibility upon the workers of the Matrimandir because of the special feature of the Matrimandir. Would you say that our relations to these directive, our attitudes, have any relation to the financial crisis and the slowing up of work – the blockage, really – in work and money?

I don't know about this 'attitude', but it is a direct result of the failure of the general consciousness to rise up to the required level. The crisis is one of consciousness and not of money. If individuals take pains and build up the type of consciousness that is expected of them, things are bound to change.

Does this mean that each individual, in a close-knit community like this does his own yoga, works upon himself?

Both, simultaneously.

Upon the community as well?

The first priority is the individual yoga and based upon that comes the contribution to the collective development. If you are not enlightened yourself, there is little that you can meaningfully contribute to the general progress. So the individual development is the basis; contribution to the collectivity is the result.

Today in this time of crisis, so much emphasis is being laid upon the gathering of the money force. Can we take your word that it is actually a crisis of consciousness?

You see they would say that to develop your consciousness you must first have your body; you have to live. I agree that living in the physical world and having a physical body, the first thing necessarily is to keep the physical body alive. Whatever is necessary we have to do it — it's not the main thing, but it has to be done. Just as we devote a certain part of our day for our physical needs, though we do not attach importance to it, but still they are indispensable, aren't they? Similarly to find the ways and means to keep our body and soul together somebody has to organise it all. One needn't attach too much importance to it but it has to be done. Mother tried to see that that problem did not pose itself; the inmates did not have to do that. That was Mother's central idea, that it would be provided. If only you have the goodwill, the aspiration, you will be given the means wherewith you can build the City of Truth. For various reasons, things did not work out or they have not worked out yet — it is not that they can't work it out or they won't. The same problem as in the Ashram is here, that is all. But I suppose it will be easier to solve here because of the fewer numbers here.

Also, in meeting a problem there's chance to raise one's consciousness.

Yes. It all depends, ultimately, upon the spirit with which we work out the progress. If we do that as part of our collective yoga, to provide means for everyone around us to live a healthy life in order to participate in the experiment or project, it does become something more than an administrative measure.

The question boils down to this: each individual has to look into himself and see what has been his contribution, positively and negatively. That will be a more rewarding process. Have I by my thought, words or actions contributed to a general disharmony at any time? Have I made any sacrifice for the collective good? Have I given up my self-centredness? These are the lines on which the pursuit of self-inquiry has to proceed.

19

Vijnana or Gnosis

Having completed the three stages of ascent of the Soul, namely the physical, the vital and the mental, we have now come in our discussion to the stage of transition, a radical transition from the lower triple existence into the higher belt of a diviner existence. As we observed earlier, between the lower triple existence and the higher triple existence of Existence, Consciousness and Bliss, there is the link-world, the world of Truth-Knowledge. To ascend into it marks a radical departure from our lower human nature, into a divine nature. All that has gone before changes its character; what happens hereafter cannot be compared with what has gone before. Even the highest heights of the mind cannot give an idea of the realms that are beyond the mind. Sri Aurobindo observed that the top-most summits of the mind, including the overmind, still labour under this mighty shadow of ignorance, the shadow of division. It is only after you register an ascent beyond the overmental level and enter into the region of the Truth-Knowledge, that you are at last freed from the pursuing taint of ignorance and division.

This principle, the principle of the Soul's poise here — the universal Soul's poise along with its characteristic nature, is called the *Vijnana.* In Sanskrit, the Vijnana means knowledge par excellence. It is not to be identified with the same term as used in Buddhist philosophy where it means discriminative reason, pure intelligence. In Sanskrit Vijnana is something else; the principle is different. Nor is it to be confused, based upon the conception — based indeed upon spiritual experience — in the Vedanta which speaks of a massed, illumined consciousness. It is called Chaitanyaghana or Chit-ghana in the Upanishads, whereby they mean a luminous consciousness, massed around one idea, one truth of Oneness. It does not admit in its fold the truth of multiplicity.

Neither of these constitutes the truth of Vijnana. Keeping this in mind, it is profitable to compare the workings of the mind — including its farthest ranges — with the working and the functioning of the Vijnana, which we shall call for our purpose the principle of Truth-Knowledge.

The mind seeks for knowledge; it depends largely upon the report of the senses — in fact the mind itself is called the sixth sense. The five senses pursue their object, alight upon it and bring back the report to the presiding mind. The mind bases itself upon the percepts of the senses and arrives at its concepts. By the interweaving of the percepts of the senses and the concepts of the reason, the mind arrives at a certain knowledge. After arriving at that knowledge, it compares its knowledge with other knowledge similarly arrived at. It draws upon memory, it draws upon inference, analyses, synthesises, judges. But with all these processes it arrives at something which at best is a tentative knowledge. The knowledge of today is always replaceable when a larger knowledge dawns tomorrow. But the way of the Truth-Mind, the Truth-Knowledge is quite different. It does not seek for knowledge from outside. It is one with the object of knowledge. Whatever it chooses to know, this Truth-Mind knows by a sort of identity. Just as I know that I am so and so, I know what is happening in me; I know when I feel joy, I know when I feel anger. Similarly, by an equally authentic and valid experience, this Truth-Mind knows everything it chooses to know. It does not have to infer, it does not have to draw upon a past memory. All knowledge stands mapped out in its vision. The knowledge of the Vijnana is one of self-vision. It is a vision which widens itself, elongates itself as the need may be and the knowledge is delivered without having to reason it out.

Some distant idea of the working of this faculty can be got by the working of what is called Intuition. Normally what we call intuition is not intuition at all, but a vague and weak reflection of it. Man is normally accustomed to work by his logical reason and arrive at a conclusion. At times, however, the intellect is quickened and it leaps over certain steps and arrives at a conclusion which has a certainty about it, and we call that intuition. But it is only a precipitation of the working of the labouring reason. If one were to trace it back, conscientiously, one would know which were the steps that were leaped over.

This precipitation is not intuition, but a pale imitation of intuition. A truer idea of what the intuition is can be got by an observation of what is called instinct at the animal level. Animals do not have the reasoning capacity but guide themselves instinctively. They desist from eating certain leaves, they hesitate to place their feet on certain spots and so on. When there is danger, they instinctively feel its presence. This faculty is an expression of the original intuition at the animal level in a form that suits the development of that consciousness. It is interfered with when the vital mind and the reasoning mind step in.

True intuition goes straight to the solution. It is only afterwards that we may verify it. And when it comes, there is such a sense of self-evident authenticity about that there can be no mistaking it. But even this intuition is not a direct working of the Truth-Mind or the Supramental Consciousness. It is only what Sri Aurobindo calls an edge; an edge of light, a ray, proceeding from the light of the Gnosis. For our purpose Vijnana, Truth-Knowledge, the Supramental and the Gnosis are the same.

When there is an intuition, the human mind rushes in and mixes its own stuff with it so that ultimately what we have, even when the intuition is pure enough in its origin, is a mixed or a pseudo-intuition. To be free from this intrusion,

Sri Aurobindo points out, we have to take care to keep out the mixture of physical mentality which always depends for its knowledge upon appearances, the vital mentality which is moved largely by desires, emotions, passions, preferences and the limited mind which is always governed by its pet notions, prejudices, likes and dislikes. All these three are distorting elements which insist on mixing themselves with the intuitive light. These three, Sri Aurobindo recalls, are the three knots which have to be loosened by invoking the grace of the Supreme. To that we shall come later.

When the intrusion of these lower workings of the mind, of the pseudo-working of a coated intuition are checked, one ascends in consciousness. One has to cross through level after level — the level of illumination, the level of inspiration, the level of intuition — before one is admitted into the realm of the Gnosis, the world of Light, the world of Truth-Power.

The first distinguishing characteristic of this truth principle is that knowledge is invariably accompanied by power. It does not happen here as it happens on other levels that there is an idea, but the idea cannot effectuate itself for want of a supporting power. Here, Truth reveals itself as Knowledge and that Knowledge carries its own self-effectuating Power. It is not even a combination; it is a double principle of Knowledge and Power. To put it in other words, it is a creative truth. The ancients had a way of speaking in picturesque symbols; they spoke of this Vijnana, this principle, as the glorious Sun of Truth, of whom the physical sun on our planet is only a symbol. This Sun they also called the Eye of the Gods, because the functioning is through vision. Whoever attains that level, sees with that vision and not with the borrowed light passing through the physical organ of the eye, which can be deformed by any defect in the instrument. It is a self-seeing eye of light. It is also called the creator or the manifestor of the universe because the Truth that shines through the Sun of Truth is creative. That is why it is called the creative Sun, the releaser, the manifestor, the creator. On the highest levels, even on the overmind, one gets only the rays of this Supramental Sun. One does not live directly in the light. And as you know, the principle of the Overmental creation is multiplicity, though based upon unity. Each one pursues its independent career. There are three stages, of which Sri Aurobindo speaks, through which we have to pass before we can rise to our full stature in the Gnosis.

The first stage is the marshalling of the rays — there is the Sun with its million rays extended. The seeker, as he ascends, prays to the godhead to help him to marshall these rays which are so many thoughts, so many ideas, so many truths that are visible. They all have to be brought together in the order of their relation, arranged in the order of the Truth. That is the first step. After these rays are marshalled, arranged, they are to be gathered together and fused in the body of the Sun. Once all these diversities and multiplicities, which are signified by the rays of the Sun, are unified, are fused in the body of the luminous orb, the Truth reveals itself. That is the goodliest form of all, the fairest form of Thee where all is seen in the orb of the creative Truth, all is seen as manifestations of the One. And the climax comes when the Being in the Sun is realised as none other than I. This is the great cry of the Upanishads, the marvellous discovery of the seer when he realises, at the end of his journey to the Truth-world, that not only is the whole universe contained in the Truth that he sees, but he and that Truth are One. So himself, the world and the creative Person are all one. This is the climactic experience of ascent into the Gnosis.

I spoke of the vedic parable in which there is reference to the three knots. The legend dates some 5,000 years ago, and a legend in the past traditions always clothed some significant truths. The story goes that there was a king, and he had no son to succeed him on to the throne. So he prayed to god Varuna, the god of vastness, purity, the god presiding over the ocean, for a son. And when he prayed, he said, "Give me progeny and I will sacrifice the first son to you."

The god was obliging and he did get a son, but the king conveniently forgot his promise. But the god would not let him forget; he afflicted him with dropsy. The story of the broken promise got round and the son — he was hardly ten or twelve — was afraid that his father would give him up to be sacrificed. So without his father's knowledge he ran away to the forests and there, in the course of his wanderings, he came across a poor couple who were starving. They had a son. The prince struck a bargain with them that their son, called Shunashepha, would be given in exchange for a hundred head of cattle. The bargain was struck; the young boy, younger than the prince, was brought to the palace, the cattle were exchanged and a huge ceremony was started with Shunashepha tied to the stake with strings in three places, top, middle and below. When the ceremony was in progress and hymns were being recited to propitiate the deity, a sage took pity on the young boy and told him to invoke that very deity with a particular hymn. And the story goes that the boy went on invoking, in fifteen verses, and praying to the god in the most significant verse to release him from those three knots so that he could once again look upon the face of his Mother, the Infinite.

Western scholars interpret this hymn as an evidence of human sacrifice. As usual they are far off the mark. This is a parable of the human soul tied to the stake of Ignorance. The name Shunashepha, in its derivative sense, means a ray of delight. The human soul issues from the creative delight of the Supreme. Each soul is a ray of Bliss. Here, in this field of ignorance, in this world of ignorance that is enveloped in darkness, by obscurity, the soul is triply bound to the lower nature. The lowermost bondage is the physical bondage; the middle is the bondage of the vital with its passions, ambitions, desires; and the higher bondage is the mind. So these are the three bondages that the human soul wants to be delivered of with the aid of the grace of God, so that it can look again on the face of its Mother, who is the infinity, Aditi — the Mother of the gods, the Mother of all, Aditi, whom Sri Aurobindo describes as the vast infinite taking a form.

This is the parable of the human soul. Before one is admitted to the sanctum of the Truth-Mind, these three knots must be dissolved. What Mother calls the triple ego — the ego of the physical, the ego of the vital and the most difficult, the ego of the mental. The Veda does not speak of cutting the knots, but of loosening, untying them very much in the line of Mother's thought. She too doesn't believe in surgical methods but in loosening, untying the knots.

This Vedic parable is repeated in the life of each and every individual at some stage or other in the course of his evolutionary journey to the Spirit. Just as the legendary crucifixion of Christ is repeated in each individual case before man is admitted into the penetralia of the Divine, similarly is the resolution of the three bonds in the hall of Death.

Could you say a little more about the name Shunashepha?

It means Ray of Bliss, of which human joy is a deformation.

Could you explain the difference between cutting the knots and untying the knots?

The knots in the lower nature are formed in the long course of evolution due to involvement in ignorance and obscurity and the fact of our being rooted in the inconscience. So this has developed certain convolutions and knots. The old Indian — not the ancient but the medieval Indian — way and the way of ascetic disciplines all over the world, was to make a radical decision to cut off the offending parts which were knotted, which refused to progress. So from the soul, from the central being, a decision was made and they were psychologically cut off. They were no more allowed to participate in the journey. Now the Vedic way, the Mother's and Sri Aurobindo's way, is not to shut out any part, not to cut out any section, but to patiently loosen the knots that have formed down the centuries and reset the working. Each part must be in its proper place — the proper placement of emotion, of thoughts, of ideas —at present they are all in the wrong places. When they are gathered up and put in their proper functionings the knots are loosened. In re-forming the personality, nothing is to be excised, nothing is to be cut out. All are to be gathered up, released from their clamps and permitted to play their respective parts in the journey to the Divine. It is easy enough to renounce, to leave out certain parts which are difficult and go ahead with only a little part which is awakened, which is not too much involved. Thereby, however, man forfeits the trust placed in him by the all-wise Creator.

How can the experiences of human delight, human love, be transformed in daily life to those of Divine Love and Divine Bliss?

There is some element common between Divine Love and human love; that element is to be extended, enlarged. Ignore the other elements, but deepen and cultivate that particular element which is in common with the higher love. For instance, the element in human love which expresses itself in self-giving; the question of demand in human love comes later, but the first step is to give oneself. May be between a man and a woman, between a mother and her child — it is a self-giving. This first step of self-giving is a divine movement; the human course of development is against it — aggrandisement, ego, self-taking is the root. But it is when the love begins to manifest that the first movement to give oneself — maybe a motivated love, but the fact remains that one gives oneself. Mother says to catch hold of that hook, eliminate the impure elements like motive, like a demand and a claim following the expression of love; they are the human, vitiating elements.

Separate them, go on deepening and enlarging the area of pure love. As you go on doing it you will begin to touch the fringe of Divine Love. Thereafter a stage will come when the person on whom you center your love just disappears. That power of love, that faculty of expressing in self-giving extends itself spontaneously to all around. The person who was the cause of your first exercising that faculty is no more than an excuse. Human love, individual love, acquires the character of universal love, and one step more and it stumbles into the Divine Love.

Love is a power, if only you will allow it to grow without making it a prisoner of the vital. It draws out the soul from its depths, it brings out the best in you — the nobility of the soul. That a man or a woman can sacrifice, give himself or herself without expecting anything in return is a decisive movement that links human love to the Divine. If, because human love has been associated with the lower vital, you are to reject love, the heart, the Mother warns, will turn into a dry stone. Even when the Divine comes you will be unable to respond with love. You may intellectually, mentally, conceive, receive, but the heart will be dead. The heart is a God-given place for the cultivation of love.

At the level where you are, start feeling love — for an animal, love for an idol, love for a person. "Love is the hoop of God, our hearts to combine", as Sri Aurobindo says in *Eric*. It is man's lien on the absolute; through love we lay our claim on the Divine. The origin of all creation is Love, the glorious culmination, also, will be in the blossoming of Love. When the Supramental consciousness organises itself fully on earth, the characteristic atmosphere will be one of Love, pure Love. And there is nothing that Love cannot achieve — that's why the Mother says that Love is the greatest power. Our image of it may be deformed, may be diminished, but the truth remains.

Do you know if Sri Aurobindo ever commented upon the plane that Christ lived - overmental, or whatever it be? We want to have some knowledge of the kingdom of heaven.

If we take it that the truth that Christ came to manifest or establish on earth is the truth of Love, then we cannot classify it in terms of these planes because the source of Love is not in the vertical order, but in the psychic behind the whole thing. There is love on every plane. There are certain manifestations which cannot be evaluated in terms of planes. When they derive from the soul — like Delight, like Love — they are present on each plane. So all that we can say is that his was a spiritual consciousness. Christ came to manifest not only spiritual Love but to establish the fact of Grace, that the Divine Grace alone can save man.

20

Conditions of Attainment to the Gnosis

It would be useful if we rapidly go over the topic we discussed when we last met. The topic was the Gnosis, or the Supramental world. We studied the precise place of this world of Gnosis in the gradation of the evolutionary stairs and saw that it is the link-world between our lower hemisphere — the physical, the vital, the mental worlds, ending with the higher overmental summits — and the higher hemisphere of the worlds of Saccidananda; Existence, Consciousness, and Bliss. It is this link-world that makes the lower hemisphere a projection of the higher. It is that which works out the will and intention of the creative Saccidananda in the universe that is under manifestation.

We also saw that it is a world where knowledge is spontaneous. One does not have to labour in the manner of the logical mind, because all knowledge is there self-contained; it is knowledge by identity, not by reasoning. It is also a world which opens out on its summit to the vastitude of Delight and Bliss, for the worlds of Ananda, Bliss, are the first to greet us when we rise beyond the highest mental and overmental levels. Thereafter come the worlds of Consciousness, sheer awareness, which in turn lead to the Infinite Existence which is a sheer Existence.

Now, the topic for our discussion today deals with the conditions for reaching this world of Gnosis. Organised as it is on totally different principles, one has to equip oneself with the necessary psychological frame, state of consciousness, that can contact and that can enter into the portals of the world of Gnosis.

In the mental world we have seen that the dominant power is one of mental intelligence. It is not that that is the only power operative in the mental world. On every plane, there is one characteristic power which rules, which dominates, and all the other six of the total seven powers subserve it. But the world gets its name by the dominant power that rules it. Mental intelligence is the characteristic power of the mental world. Nothing registers in the mental being unless it is cognised, interpreted and assimilated by the mental intelligence. The instrumentation of the physical senses is not there as in our physical world, here. But the mental world has its own subtle, mental senses which grasp the object and report to the mental intelligence; all told, it is a mental operation and the presiding power is the mental intelligence.

Man, here on earth, is also a mental being, but he is not the mental being who lives in the mental world proper. He is here involved in physical matter, living physical matter. That is why his mental apparatus is not at its highest; it is always clogged, always dependent upon the physical instrumentation. He has to depend for data — at any rate in the beginning — on the physical senses that make an impact, contact things and movements, report to the cognising mind, the analysing mind which notes these reports of the physical senses, arrives at its own conclusions and stamps them as knowledge. Whether what is so arrived at is real knowledge, half-knowledge or false knowledge is another matter. All these questions, however, do not obtain when once we go to the level of the Gnosis. There, knowledge does not have to be gathered. There there is a vast principle and power of knowledge which functions automatically, spontaneously. A Gnostic being has only to will what he wants to know and there is an immediate welling up of the knowledge, or a revelation of what is to be known. That is because the knowledge that rules as consciousness on this plane is all-pervading; it is inherent and it contains the contents of everything which it chooses to know.

In the traditional yoga of Patanjali — Rajayoga as it is called — there is a technical expression, *samyama*, concentration. If you concentrate enough and with sufficient force on a particular object, that object yields its contents to you. In Rajayoga it is a *siddhi*, an accomplishment arrived at by yogic effort; but in the Gnostic world it is an effortless unveiling of knowledge. In order, however, to arrive at that state of consciousness where knowledge is self-evident, a most important condition has first to be fulfilled. That condition is to dispossess oneself of the deforming load of the ego. One has to discard the separative walls of the ego. As long as one has the consciousness that one is separate, feels that all the others are others, and lives shut up in one's own separative formation, it is impossible to get through the portals of the Gnostic world.

Mother has said a hundred times and more that unless we break up our limited egoistic formations and breathe a larger consciousness, learn to identify ourselves more and more with the universe, it is idle to expect that we can touch the Supermind. It is impossible for the Supermind to make a direct entry into a person who is still breathing the tainted air of egoism. To put it in other words, before you can become a Superman, you have to become a universal man. Some may call it the cosmic man, some, universal man, some the no-man, in the sense of a not-egoistic man. There is no way of bypassing this requirement. One has to identify oneself with and embrace the whole universe in his consciousness. How to cultivate this poise? First you conceive of it mentally, imagine it, accustom your thinking to the conception, regulate your day-to-day life at every level in the light of the knowledge that you and I are one with all, your interests are their interests, their interests are yours. Or to put it in the language that Sri Aurobindo has used elsewhere, unless my heart throbs with the beats of other hearts, the second step of spiritual transformation is not complete.

As we have known and discussed before, the first step is the realisation of the individual divine, what is called psychicisation. The second step is universalisation. It is only after these two capital and indispensable steps have been completed that there is the possibility of the third step of Supramentalisation, leading to its inevitable consequence of total transformation.

To come back to our theme, one has to have a real and concrete sense of unity with the universe and be totally free from the sense of separativity from others before one can breathe the air of the Gnostic world. In the Gnostic world knowledge is spontaneous; it has another feature — it is always accompanied by will, power. What happens in our terrestrial world is that when there is an idea, the necessary power to effectuate is not there and where there is some power it is blind. It does not have the necessary light, the conception, to lead it into effective action. Besides, there is the clash of one idea with another, one will with another. In the Gnostic world, these vitiations, deviations are absent. Knowledge is power, power that is will, conscious will is power; both are, as it were, two sides of the same coin. Where knowledge leads, power follows; where power manifests, knowledge supports. So it is a fulfillment of the twin powers in creation, of knowledge and light, light and power, knowledge and will.

The one condition to realise this state is that one must have the consciousness of infinity. Not limitation, but a boundless expansion. The infinity, again, is not to be conceived only as an infinite extension, as a borderless extension. It is that, of course, but it is also an infinity within, an infinity above, an infinity below. So much so that the individual feels that he is but a point, — not a negligible point of course — but a point, may be a necessary point, for the concentration of individualised action. Even infinity needs to focus itself at a point for a particular action. The individual realises that he is the point of centralisation, a point of convenience for the action of the Infinity. He is, and yet he is not, an individual. He is not in the sense with which we are familiar here, but he is because he continues to play his part as one ray of the sun. There is knowledge, there is power, there is an unmixed, unadulterated Bliss. When the consciousness is freed from the deforming element, a mixture of egoism, desire, falsehood, it feels the throb of the underlying Bliss. This Bliss is always there, but in our conditions of ignorance and limitation, it is rendered in the incomplete terms of pleasure, pain, indifference. All these are superficial renderings which it is possible to reject even in certain states of purified spiritual consciousness. One does not have to wait till one reaches the Gnostic level, but there it is natural. The Bliss that flows is irresistible. There are the seas of Delight and Ananda of which Sri Aurobindo speaks.

The whole being, at every level — level of existence, level of dynamis, will, level of knowledge, level of experience of delight — becomes a vehicle of the living Supreme. The individual no more feels that he is even an instrument, that he even reflects something. He feels he is just a centre through which almighty, creative being knows, wills, delights, exists. This is the acme of experience that a mental man, arriving and living in the Gnostic plane can experience. The conditions are, as we have seen, total elimination of ego, displacement of the reasoning and logical mind, — firstly by the silent spiritual mind opening up to the higher spiritual planes of illumination, inspiration, revelation, and intuition, — the elimination of desire and self-will. One starts in the very beginning, indeed, surrendering these loads, these vestiges from the animal past, but one's surrender reaches its culmination only when one qualifies for entry into the Gnostic world.

Any questions?

Can one attain the Gnostic world by opening up the higher levels of the mental consciousness?

Theoretically, it should be possible to attain to the Gnostic world by the opening up of the higher levels of the mental consciousness, but it would be a long and arduous effort. When the psychic is awakened, it releases many forces which break up the walls of ignorance and falsehood and facilitate the purification of the mind and the emotions, link up the lower being with the higher at its own level, and whether the mind is developed or not, the psychic forms its own channel of communication, and by love and the action of surrender which is so natural and spontaneous to it, it builds the bridge to the Gnosis.

The easiest way, the most effective way to reach the Gnostic world, the Gnostic consciousness is to find the psychic key, open the psychic realm — the heart — deepen the consciousness, go deep and deep within, allow the psychic to psychicise the whole being so that the entire system aspires in chorus for the harmonies of the Gnosis.

If the higher knowledge is above, is it useful to try to bring it into the mind by, for instance, formulating it in terms of the intellect and expressing it in words?

The fact is that one who is stationed on levels above the mind realises that all the knowledge that one has cannot be rendered in terms of the intellect. But it is possible to use the mental language, especially the symbolic aspect of it, to express the higher knowledge. But knowledge need not be always expressed in mental terms.

What I meant is, is it useful for the development of the mind to bring that higher level to the mind?

For an integral development, it is useful to develop all

the parts in the mould of the Gnostic knowledge and consciousness. Mind, being the most developed part, has the first claim to be so developed. The love and the delight aspect of it floods the heart; the knowledge and the wisdom irradiate the mind; the immutable, the immortal existence suffuses itself in the physical. One does not have to make an effort once one is stationed there firmly — these actions go on simultaneously and spontaneously. It is, of course, understood that there is always the stress of the temperament and the nature of the individual. If one has been an intellectual, a mentally developed being, there will necessarily be a preponderance of the manifestation of knowledge in that individual. In others it may be a dynamic overflow of love and delight. The way is not to build the mind in the mould of the Gnostic knowledge, but to lay it open for the higher knowledge to act upon and fill itself in the mind.

The transformation of consciousness that we're all aspiring to receive is happening all over the world, isn't it? A letter has just been received from a young man; it was addressed to "Matrimandir, Ashram Auroville" - which is very interesting. He says he's practised yoga, read a little of Indian philosophy, also Sri Ramana Maharshi's teachings and two books by Krishnamurti. He says, "I'm greatly impressed, particularly by Krishnamurti because he speaks in nowadays language and he doesn't make me believe in ideas such as a personal God in which I cannot believe. I think that I'm changing all the time, but I haven't really *changed. Even if it be better now, it is still bad. I want to find something true, something really true. I really don't know what to do.*

They say that Truth is everywhere, in each thing and in everyone, but I want to come to Auroville, so please answer if it is possible if I could get an invitation to come there, I would earn enough money to come, but without invitation, I haven't the incentive."

I think this is something that would be for you to handle.

He is from which country?

Poland.

His confusion is very understandable for he has been reading three kinds of literature, that of Ramana Maharshi, of Krishnamurti and Sri Aurobindo, hasn't he? Now each one approaches the Reality from a different angle. Krishnamurti, no doubt, speaks the modern language, but his role is one of destruction. He breaks down all the traditional constructions, the mental constructions that have grown down the ages — superstitions, mental ideas which give certain comfort to the ignorant mind by assuring it that we are safe, this is right, this will protect us, this is knowledge, and so on. His role appears to be, in the larger occult economy of things, to clear the passage, to break down all these impermanent barricades that bar the development of the mind. And those who have taken only that much help from him have been fortunate. But he says that to demolish what has been built, to de-condition the mind is enough. Thereafter there is an automatic perception of the Reality. That is, in brief, his approach.

So what has happened is that a lot of youngsters, not only in Europe, but in America and India, took enthusiastically to this approach, but afterwards found themselves rudderless. Their props were knocked down, but the Reality of which Krishnamurti speaks as being self-evident once the de-conditioning is done did not reveal itself. To him, in some way it is there because he has arrived at the frontiers of the silent mind and feels the presence of something which you can't describe. But the others who follow his instructions are left hanging in mid-air because they are not ready in their consciousness to perceive that Reality. So there is a sense of progress, but no sense of certainty.

Ramana Maharshi's teaching, which consists in asking oneself, "Who am I?" is a relentless process of self-introspection. If one sincerely does it, one gets released from the surface activity of the sense mind, but not the reasoning mind. There is, again, a sense of movement within, a feeling of progress, a certain peace which one gets as one withdraws from the frothy surface, but unless the grace of the Guru is there to push one further, it is extremely difficult to arrive at the Self that is deep within.

So in either case he has trodden the path, arrived somewhere, but not far enough. This path, if he takes to it now, will help him a good deal because he has already got the preliminary self-training — silencing the mind, dispossessing the mind of all its notions, withdrawing from the surface activity and interiorising the consciousness, looking towards the Self within. These are all of great advantage in any yoga but particularly in our yoga. So such persons should be encouraged to study more of Sri Aurobindo's works, especially his *Letters on Yoga* and the *Synthesis*.

In building that image within, focussing the imagination so that the Reality grows within, is that an image of Light, of lighted substance? Mother speaks of it in the Prayers and Meditations *as the highest and purest Light.*

It depends on oneself. Some who are used to visual experience would conceive of it or imagine it as a splendour or a radiant light. Some who have the habit of feeling would think of it as a presence. At any rate, till one has the experience, one can begin by constructing mentally that experience. That creates a certain climate, a certain groove for the experience to flow along. It also acts as a sort of magnet. Those who are fortunate are given at the very step some peep into that world, some kind of experience. They do not need to visualise, they do not need to imagine, they do not need to dream. For us, to whom what Sri Aurobindo says or Mother says has an authentic ring, to read is enough. What they have written — their remembrance, their recollection is quite enough to establish the link. But for an outsider it is only information. For those of us who are open to Sri Aurobindo and the Mother, who are linked with them in consciousness, it is a power; for the rest it is a book of philosophy or yoga. They have to resort to all kinds of mental gymnastics. In all these books on yoga published in Europe or America you are taught what you have to do step by step. You follow points one, two, three, four and hope they will lead you to a revelation. When you start doing this yoga, there is none of this step-by-step action.

I get books from various journals; they are written by people who came to India, lived under certain great masters and learnt something. On the plea that they have to deliver the goods to the Western mind, they mathematise what they have learnt. That does not work. Yoga is a natural process. The mind becomes the prisoner of a system when you follow such methods.

21

The Higher and the Lower Knowledge

We have seen the goal of the yoga of knowledge as propounded by Sri Aurobindo, the goal of the gnostic consciousness leading to a status in the bliss consciousness. In fact the peaks of the gnostic consciousness fade into the heights or the seas of bliss. Starting from matter, material life, Sri Aurobindo has shown how the human consciousness can culture itself, grade by grade, assimilate the gains of each level and ascend the ladder of existence till it reaches the gnostic levels bordering on the worlds of Ananda, Bliss. And the aim, he has made sufficiently clear, is not only to realise and possess the Divine, but also to be possessed by the Divine. One realises the objective, one realises God, not somewhere beyond but here on earth, in the circumstances of material life. Here in the field of ignorance and evolution the divine is to be realised and possessed.

The Divine is realised in this path not only in one aspect. One realises the Divine as the Impersonal, the vast impersonality that defies definition. But one also realises the Divine in his multiple personalities. Similarly, one realises the Divine in utter static passivity of poise, as also in the dynamic outpourings of his being. One realises the Divine as calm, as peace — not a static peace, but a powerful, potent peace — and equally in the multifarious activity which characterises this manifestation of God.

Secondly, one opens oneself to the Divine Consciousness, to the divine Being, and allows oneself to be filled with the successive descents of God. Simultaneously, one lifts oneself from the lower to the next higher level. Whether it is the physical body or the life-force or the thought mind or the higher levels of consciousness, one is continuously at work making the grades in the ladder of spiritual consciousness, integrating in oneself what has gone before and what is attained at present, with an eye to the future. There is a continuous process of assimilation, of reflection, and a process of identification with the Divine — the Divine everywhere, the Divine in all aspects, the Divine descending and oneself ascending into the heights of the Divine. These are the broad lines of the scheme worked out in the yoga of knowledge.

We have not touched so far on one important distinction that is in the process of the yoga of knowledge. I have once before told you that one of the ancient Upanishads speaks of two kinds of knowledge, the higher knowledge and the lower knowledge. It describes all the sixty-four arts and sciences known to intellectual man as constituting the higher knowledge, and that by which the Divine, the Immutable is known, by knowing which all else is known, as the higher knowledge.

What the ancients thought of the ultimate value of the several branches of lower knowledge will be evident to you if I once again recall to you the legend in one of the Upanishads which, I believe I have recounted to you once or twice before. The sage Narada, the divine Singer, approached the divine manifestation called Sanatkumara and told him that he had mastered all the branches of learning open to man but he had not been able to cross the ocean of sorrow in spite of it. He was reminded by the divine teacher that what he knew were only the names of things, not the Reality. What he knew were only the labels, and stressing the sheer inadequacy of the learning that he had, the teacher, so the legend goes, communicated to him the knowledge that led him across the sea of ignorance to the other shore.

Now Sri Aurobindo does not dismiss the various branches of the lower knowledge superciliously. As everywhere, he gives due weight to what has been evolved, to what has been useful, and while pointing out their limitations, he takes care to affirm their utility at their level. Speaking in this context of the various branches of the lower knowledge, — art, science, psychology, philosophy, ethics and so on — Sri Aurobindo describes how they are the starting points for the seeker. Any science, if it is honestly pursued is bound to lead to the Reality, at any rate to the gates of the Reality. He describes how physical science, by which the modern man swears, has now come to the end of its tether in its honest pursuit of truth and is face to face with a reality that it cannot comprehend, that it cannot explain; it is on the borders of the Infinite. Similarly, art opens the inner eye of man to beauty, to the aesthetic values in nature, subtilises his emotions, and prepares him for a subtler life. Psychology, the science of the mind, comes to a stage when it stands face to face with certain phenomena which it is unable to explain on its own basis — it develops into parapsychology. Parapsychology, again, leads to the borders of mysticism. Philosophy speaks of the principles of things, and a number of philosophies emphasising the different principles of things lead the seeker, the honest student, to the perception of the Principle of principles. And so on.

Take history for example. One studies the events that have happened in the life of humanity, one traces a line of development and whatever the checks and temporary setbacks one sees a forward advance of consciousness and one is forced to admit a direction, a teleology in the course of the evolutionary movement.

Each branch of learning, each limb of the knowledge called the lower knowledge has its utility. As long as man needs to be educated by these sciences and brought up to a level where he is ready to receive the higher knowledge, their role is indispensable. That is why in his voluminous writings, Sri Aurobindo has dealt with the fundamentals of the various sections of human knowledge, polity, sociology, culture, philosophy, mysticism, and so on. But everywhere he takes care to point out that these sciences and arts approach the Reality from outside. At their best they can expose the processes of things, how things happen. To the extent that the processes lend themselves to the human eye and the human intelligence, they explain. They perceive something of the Reality from across a veil, the veil of the senses, but they also tend towards the Reality.

It is when all that the lower knowledge has to provide has been provided that the stage arrives for the higher knowledge to be attempted. And the means to realise the higher knowledge of God, of the Divine Reality in its manifold aspects, is through yoga. Yoga is a discipline — you may call it an art, a science, but a deeper art and a higher science — which aims to link the soul, one's own being, with the Reality directly. It doesn't approach from outside but directly, and there are three ways by which yoga attempts to arrive at the consummation of the higher knowledge which is the direct realisation of the divine Reality.

The first way is purification. It doesn't need to be emphasised that in the normal working of our mind and senses there is so much impurity — likes and dislikes, prejudices, preferences, conscious and unconscious — that perverts, that misleads the senses into getting distorted reports that influence the mind to judge in a biased way. When we speak of impurity in yoga, it is not so much the physical impurities, but the psychological impurities that are meant. When people speak of purification and ask about purification through food, external purification, things are not put in their proper perspective. Of course external cleanliness is necessary, a certain amount of purity in physical food is necessary, but what is more important is the psychological purity. Even in food, mind you, it is the psychological purity that is emphasised in the Indian tradition.

There are many stories that I could tell you about how yogis have suffered on account of the impure thoughts that had passed through the mind of the person who had either cooked the food or served it. You are all probably aware of the incident in the life of Ramakrishna Paramahamsa. He was an unassuming man. One day he went to the house of one of his rich disciples. There all were served some rice cakes. There were a number of people, and the head of the house had them served first and then he himself went to attend upon the other guests of his social class. As soon as the saint touched the rice cake he got a burning sensation in the whole body and he started shivering. He didn't allow his disciples to make a fuss, but he quietly slipped out. He later explained that someone in the household connected with the food must have had impure thoughts. And thereafter it was verified and confirmed.

Similarly, I have known of many instances in the Mother's life when impurities in the activities or in the minds of devotees and disciples in the Ashram have had a deleterious effect upon her body. Once when she was found scratching her arms on the playground, someone asked her what was the matter for she was not known to scratch like that. She just replied, "Someone is indulging in sex". Another incident: as you know, Mother was taking very little solid food for many years. She used to take only a little grape juice in the morning for breakfast — a very small tumblerful. Once it happened that when the grapes arrived they were kept in a basin under the tap for washing and the man in charge just happened to go inside for something. At the time two of our boys passed by. They looked at the grapes and said, "What fine grapes!" That was all. When the juice of these grapes was served the next day to the Mother, she did not touch it. She had not been told anything but still her being was repelled by food tainted by the passing desire of the boys. Those boys had not meant anything; they could not help themselves. But this is the reason why one emphasises psychological purity in spiritual life much more than physical purity.

The first step, as I have said, in trying to attain to the higher knowledge, in opening oneself to the higher knowledge, is purification; purification of the mind, purification of the nerves, purification of the subtle body. Each one has its different technique — perhaps we will come to it sometime later. Next comes concentration. Everyone knows how our faculties are spread in a hundred directions. We are not aware that we are spread out in so many diverse directions. Concentration consists in gathering all our faculties, movement, thought, emotions gradually, and with a will, focussing them and fixing them on one object. It is only by this process of a compulsive marshalling of our faculties and focussing them on the object of our pursuit that we can establish a link with the object and force the object to yield its content to our perceiving, receptive, grasping consciousness.

As one is purified, as the consciousness is concentrated and settled upon the Reality, or an aspect of the Reality, there is an effortless reflection in that consciousness of that Reality in the quietude of our being. Like the moon reflected in placid waters, to take an image from the Upanishads. When this reflection is complete, when this concentration is at its premium, one attains a complete identification with the Reality. One is no more aware of a division, of a separation between oneself and the Divine.

This is the object of higher knowledge. Higher knowledge is that which reveals the divine Reality in oneself, establishes an identification, and makes one one with it. We have said that the Divine so realised, at any rate in this context, is not the Alone but the Divine manifest in the universe, in all its powers, in all its values, at all levels. The

Divine is realised in himself, in oneself, in all things around. This is the object of the higher knowledge to which the lower knowledge prepares the way.

The Mother has described in many of her talks how it is indispensable for the mind to be educated, to be cultured in the ways of the intellect. The intellect does not give the final answer but it has to be stimulated. The intelligence has to be made dynamic, active, and as the brain is being developed by effort, new cells are formed and new grooves form themselves into which the higher knowledge can flow. The lower knowledge has a great use, and the higher knowledge, when it dawns, does not reject the lower avenues. It makes them part of itself, suffuses the lower branches of knowledge with its own light and makes them so many windows or gateways of approach to the mission of the Lord.

Any questions?

Can we get help from the Mother now that she has left her body?

Your question reminds me of a cynical remark made by someone "Now Mother is nobody's property." Actually the opposite is true, everybody has access to her. Everyone can talk to her, refer to her. She has given herself to everyone. Not only here, but even abroad. I have received letters from Rome, from Holland and from other countries saying it was never so easy to contact her. They have only to think of the Mother to feel her presence, to get the definite word of guidance. An old lady in Rome was told in a vivid vision, "This is not the time to weep. Look!" And, she said, the floodgates of joy were opened. That was on the 18th of November 1973.

I suppose it is self-evident that when Mother cast off the physical vesture, her consciousness spread wide and, in this case, it is an act of Grace. She has deliberately held herself at the disposal of her children. Only yesterday someone who had a certain inner contact with the Mother all these years told me that when she looked within she was told "I have deliberately held myself here. Now I have to spread out."

I would like to open a topic that is connected with Matrimandir. When Matrimandir is completed, Mother has said there will be no photographs, no flowers, no incense in it. In view of this, what is your view of the offering of flowers and incense and the presence of photographs in the construction of the Matrimandir?

As long as it helps us to make the Presence concrete to ourselves, it can be continued. When the whole structure is complete, when the full Presence installs itself, all these things will be irrelevant. By that time we also will have developed enough not to need them. But I think that at this stage we do need the support of visual representations, of the purifying vibrations of incense of which Mother speaks so highly in *Prayers and Meditations*. They have a great occult significance. They drive away and discourage little elementals, little hostile spirits from establishing themselves in the atmosphere. Inertia, sloth, mischief, falsehood — these are discouraged in the presence of light, in the presence of incense, in the presence of a photograph or something which radiates vibrations of a higher consciousness. If we can evolve such vibrations from within ourselves, then nothing else will be necessary. But are we always in that condition? We don't live within ourselves, man doesn't live alone. He is subject to so many influences and he is not always at his best, at his highest.

These photographs are always, for us, not just images, representations, likenesses, but living symbols that put us in touch immediately with the Reality behind, with the consciousness behind. I have known Mother to explain what kind of consciousness she had when a particular photograph was taken; she attached that much importance to it and she said that any problem would disappear if one just concentrated upon it. There is a photograph taken in 1961 or 1962 in which Mother is just reclining on a couch looking. When I just saw it, I lost the sense of possessing a head, that is,

I felt as if I had no lid over my head limiting me. It was a kind of experience of the Infinite. So when I sent to her in the evening I told Mother what I had felt as soon as I saw this photograph. She laughed and said, "Yes, that is precisely the state of consciousness in which I was when the photograph was taken." Then I wanted copies of that photograph to be made and sold. It was a coloured photograph, but unfortunately the person who had the negative had spoiled it. So to make it available, I got a block made of the copy that I had, signed by the Mother, and included it as a colour print in one of my books *Lamps of Light.*

Some years later, I think ten years or so, Champaklal once spoke to Mother about that photograph, referring to it as the photo which Mother liked. This was ten years after, mind you — and people think that Mother used to forget things. Referring to the photograph Champaklal had said, "The photograph which Madhav had brought to Mother and Mother liked!" Mother said, "The photo Madhav liked!" So he came to ask me to check up. He said, "I have a recollection that Mother liked it and you had taken it to her but Mother said that it was you who liked it." I said, "Yes, Mother didn't like it."

Well, these are all sweet memories. We don't need memories to keep her living with us, but they come, they come.

In the answer that you gave regarding the role of the Matrimandir in the spiritual evolution, my notes are not clear in the part where you discussed the link that Mother established with many levels of cosmic consciousness. I will read you what I have and perhaps you could clarify it.

> "This is clear, that the Matrimandir, being a concrete expression of the Mother's consciousness-force will always stand as a reservoir of inspiration, a lighthouse radiating continually the manifestation of Truth as it has been embodied in the Mother. What Mother's embodiment has been to us here, the full-fledged Matrimandir will be to the whole of humanity."

Now this is the part about which I have a question: "In the course of her life on earth, the Mother has established links with many levels of cosmic existence . . .

I think you can end with "humanity". I think that day I must have thought something else earlier, and so the question came of the links with the different levels of consciousness. It is not so necessary. These two sentences sum up what I have said.

But this is very important for our relation to the Truth-Light of which the Matrimandir will be an instrument as a spiritual mechanism, which I think is enlightening. Because I believe you said . . .

Yes, I did say it.

. . . .not only the light and consciousness will be radiating from the Matrimandir, but also the means of realising them for each individual.

It can be there, but the mention about the links with the various levels of consciousness, I think, will be unnecessarily complicating matters there. That sentence you can remove.

So then: "What the Mother's embodiment has given us here, the full-fledged Matrimandir will be to the whole of humanity. Not only will the Truth-Light and Consciousness be radiating from the Matrimandir, but also the means of realising them?"

No, wait. It is incomplete. Not only the Truth-Light and Consciousness will be radiating from the Matrimandir, but also the means of realising them *will be made living* to each individual. Is it clear? The Truth-Light and Consciousness will be radiating from the Matrimandir and the means of realising them will remain dynamic. . . .with the passage of time, they get encrusted and they lose their original force, but the Matrimandir being what it is, what she has designed it to be, they will retain their dynamism.

What is the next step in yoga?

You mean the yoga of the evolving earth-consciousness, is that right? There is a thing like the individual yoga; my yoga, her yoga, anybody's yoga. Mother was doing a yoga for the earth in evolution. She constituted herself as a representative of the evolutionary cosmic being and was pursuing a process, working out a process of transformation. She had brought it to a certain point; it has to be continued and it will be continued. As far as it can furthered on higher levels that is being done, but for that part of it which has to be done on earth, another manifestation will have to come and continue it.

Could that manifestation be the Matrimandir?

Can't say. As I visualise it, it will be another new being in a body made there, that will manifest and complete the process. Beyond what has been done now, it is not possible to do in a normally born human body.

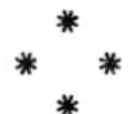

I do believe what Mother and Sri Aurobindo called the intermediate race or something like that will have to appear before supramental body proper can manifest itself on earth. An intermediate stage has to be worked out. I do believe that, though I don't have a precise formulation in my mind yet as to what form it will take.

It was hoped that this human body would transmute itself into that bridge body, that highly subtilised body which would form the transitional link between the human and the supramental, but things had to stop before that took place.

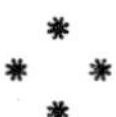

No, I don't think that this comes under the spiritistic phenomena. There are photographs I have seen in certain books of Leadbeater and Blavatsky where vague outlines of the spirits have been captured. I think that is quite different; that plane bordering on the physical plane — almost the subtle physical — which can be photographed by very sensitive film is different from the higher levels of which we speak at this time. The supramental or the intermediate plane — I think those levels are different.

There are beings of light who are helping the cosmic evolution, whom the subtle eye or the awakened psychic eye can see. But those forms are quite different from the forms and figures of the spirits which come in the mediumistic seances. One needs to have a shift of consciousness to see those forms of light. When I first came here — I believe it was in 1937, when I was nineteen, — and I was standing on the terrace here to see Mother walking on the terrace, my teacher was standing by my side. He asked me, "What do you see?" I said "Mother is walking." "What else do you see?" I said, "She has put on a gown and she is walking." "You don't see anything else?" "No" I said. Then he just touched me. "Look" he said, and immediately I saw the aura around her and as she was walking, that bluish envelope-like thing, right from the toe to some inches above her head, was continuously walking along with her. So that is what I call a shift of consciousness, whether natural or induced. That is necessary to perceive these higher forms of life.

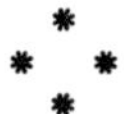

Reversal of consciousness comes at the end of a long period of effort. A long effort has to go on by willed aspiration to change, by invoking the higher grace and help. And it is when things are ready that, when we least expect it, we find there is a sudden change in the very poise, in the very direction of the consciousness. That is called the reversal of consciousness; it is the end of a process.

So the process everybody knows. We have to do it; it is a long process — a reversal of consciousness comes and stays for some time, then again the consciousness goes back to its original position. It is the conversion of consciousness that is permanent. A number of reversals of consciousness ultimately settle themselves into the conversion of consciousness. Once the conversion of consciousness is effected, there is no going back.

22

Gnosis and Ananda

We have discussed the Gnosis, described the various levels that the seeker has to ascend before he arrives at the Gnosis. The Gnosis, however, is not the end; the Supramental plane is not the terminus. It is, as we said, a link-world between the higher hemisphere and the lower hemisphere of matter, life and mind. Once you go to the level of the Gnosis, there is a complete reversal of consciousness. You arrive at the Transcendent, above the universe.

We have to remember that though the divine consciousness, the Saccidananda has its station there, in the higher hemisphere on its own, it is involved in every plane of creation. That is why it is possible to realise the Divine, to realise the Divine Bliss, Ananda, on any level that we choose. It is possible to realise it even by concentrating purely on the physical plane, because in matter, too, is the spirit.

There is a line of yoga in which you deeply scrutinise the physical body, intensify your search into matter, make your experience more and more subtle, the physical being goes into a kind of sleep, a sleep of self-concentration, or it merges into the Self that presides over the physical level, Saccidananda, the Ananda aspect in matter. Thereby one experiences a certain kind of liberation. One behaves like a child of God; the mind is not cared for, the other aspects are left out, one acts as one feels — irresponsibly from the world's point of view, but one acts in freedom. This kind of liberation that many of you have either seen or read of in India, is called the physical liberation — the realisation of God in the physical. You will find many Sannyasins, God-men, lying on ant hills, living in forests, looking so crude, so dirty, but there is a light in their eyes, there is a love in their hearts. They may throw a stone at you, but that stone may cure your disease if you go for a cure.

There are, similarly, possibilities of realising the divine Bliss on the level of life, what Bergson called the *elan vital*, the moving, the dynamic vital. One concentrates there, looks upon life as divine and arrives at a point by appropriate yoga by which the Divine is reflected in the currents of the life force. One merges into the Self of the life plane within and without. Thereby, one is liberated into a kind of freedom which throws off the yoke of both the mind and the body, and there is what Sri Aurobindo describes as the "dizzy dance of life". You will find such a one shattering to pieces all your conventions; he will express what he has gained in a wild abandon.

Similarly, it is possible to realise the Divine on the level of the mind. One realises him in thought, in ideas, in a certain detachment, rejects life as belonging to a passing moment. One takes a stand in the witness poise, merges in the Self behind, and has always a consciousness that is aloof, that is in union with the divinity that presides, that witnesses. Such a person is a hermit, a sage, a contemplative seer.

In the mind itself there are various levels. It is possible to realise the Divine in the thought-mind, the higher mind, the illumined mind and so on till you come to the level of the Gnosis. Each philosophy presents its own approach to the Divine and insists on its own way and nothing else. The integral philosophy is the one which gives due weight to every approach, to every possibility of realising the Divine on every level. It condemns none but shows the place of each in the rising tiers of creation, of manifestation, and weaves them into a pattern of rising perfection. One arrives at the Gnosis, the Supramental or the Knowledge-Will Consciousness; there also one realises the Divine Bliss as a concomitant of the Gnostic stage. The seeker that crosses into this belt is not what he was in the lower hemisphere. He is now a point, a center, for the radiation and the flow of the Divine Consciousness. The soul is not separate from Nature as in the terrestrial belt, but arrives at a certain biune poise with Nature, — the Lord and his Spouse, Ishwara and his Shakti, one and yet two, one in essence, but two in functioning, in manifestation.

When the soul arrives at this stage there is a unity, a union of the two, but a necessary polarity in manifestation. This, however, is not the end. Here the emphasis is still on the Knowledge-Will aspect of the Divine, but there is the other side — the aspect of Bliss. As one of the oldest Upanishads describes: there is the self of food, by which they mean the material self. Indwelling that material self is the self of life. Indwelling this life-self is the mental self, the mind-self; indwelling the mental self is the knowledge-self, and indwelling the knowledge-self is the Self of all the selves, the Self of Bliss. It is at the creative root of all life. That is why the world of Ananda is decribed in the Veda as the world of birth, giving birth to whole creation, its source, its fountain.

When, in the course of spiritual development, the soul crosses from the Gnostic into the Bliss world, all becomes subsidiary. Knowledge, power, movement, all become various formulations of an overwhelming Bliss. They become particular scintillations of a Bliss which is no more underlying but is overflowing. Sri Aurobindo describes how when a man arrives at this level even the aspiration for liberation falls away. He traces how the divine Creator draws men to Himself through various lures. The first lure is the lure of material comfort, of the prizes of the life-force, of the prizes of the mind, which man can earn and enjoy on earth by turning to God, by praying to God, by invoking the Grace of God. Next, for more developed people there are the lures of heaven — eternal joy, eternal happiness, undying light. Later even these fall away and there is what Sri Aurobindo calls a very subtle lure, the lure of Nirvana, the lure of escape. All is rejected and the 'I' merges into an undisturbable, immutable silence or Bliss. Sri Aurobindo points out that even this lure of wanting to escape, of wanting to be liberated, falls off when one touches the world of Bliss. For, as another Upanishad points out: when one realises the supracosmic Ananda, what is there to fear? It is only when the mind is still ignorant, when the mind is removed even a centimeter from the Bliss, from unity with the Divine, that there is fear. When one merges into the Divine Brahman, who is spread all over, there is no second — fear can come only when there is another. So with the elimination of the disease of falsehood, the yields of falsehood also go; there is neither the desire nor the striving after liberation. All becomes a movement of the Divine.

One is no more afraid to descend from that level into the world of ignorance and suffering. Ignorance and suffering have different values, they make a different impact for a man established in the Ananda consciousness. He reacts differently, for him there is no hesitation. Whether he descends, or whether he accepts to be the ascending soul, he participates freely, without bounds in the divine movement of manifestation. He is the acme of achievement for the present cycle of evolution. More there may be, and there could be, because there can be no boundaries, no finish, no finale in the Infinite. But what is intended for man in his present cycle of evolution is this summum bonum of Bliss.

Which is the Upanishad that elaborates on Bliss?

It is the Taittiriya Upanishad. It is stated: From Ananda all things are born, in Ananda they live and leaving they depart into Ananda. In the Veda it is not called the world of Bliss, it is called the world of Birth, *janaloka*. The Vedas speak of the worlds from the top. First there is the Existence, Consciousness, Birth — not Bliss — and then there is the vast world of Light, next comes the world of the mind, the world of life, the world of food, or matter. The whole conception of

Indian positive philosophy is that the whole world exists because of this undercurrent of Bliss. If there was not this underlying bliss, there could not be the will to live; and in spite of all odds man wants to live. Somewhere in *The Life Divine*, Sri Aurobindo remarks that after all is said and done, the sum total of happiness is more than the sum total of suffering and that is why man wants to live. Barring occasional aberrations like suicides, man doesn't want to die, he wants to live. There is, underlying every experience, a stream of delight. That is the delight which the Creator continously draws from His Creation and which you and I, as replicas or images of the Creator, are intended to draw. It is to draw your attention to this aspect and this possibility that the science of aesthesis concentrates on drama, poetry, epics, in describing situations which are outwardly painful and produce suffering but which in some ways draw the sap of delight in it, so that you want to sit and see it. You may shed tears, but they are tears that purify. That is because even pain and pleasure are imperfect values of an underlying bliss.

In Indian Sanskrit literature there are as many as nine "sentiments", *Rasas*, as they call them, nine forms — heroism, love, laughter, fear, disgust etc; — all these are various streams of the underlying delight of life which has to be drawn. The more cultivated a person is, the more is he able to draw the sap of delight from all experiences, even from experiences that seem contrary to an undeveloped being. That is why the creative principle is delight.

The Lord came forth in an ebullition of delight. The delight of creation, the delight of manifesting himself in conditions which are the very opposite of his own, that was the wager which the Divine took against himself. In the last chapter of *The Riddle of this World* in answer to a French questioner, Sri Aurobindo describes how this idea could have come — all was bliss, all was full, plenary consciousness, there was great delight. But a shadow came, an idea came, possibly thus: "Supposing there is no consciousness, there is apparently no existence, there is no delight. How can I manifest there?" The Divine took up the challenge; the idea came and with the idea the possibility. Then to realise the possibility the whole creation started. A million sparks went out of Him. They are we who are the souls, who are the sparks carrying out His will. And we are today in the midstage of this evolution which is climbing back to the source of Delight. It is not out of caprice that He has plunged into creation. When the consciousness which has issued from the Supreme has passed through all these movements, gathered all experiences, and then goes back it will be far richer in content than the original consciousness that came out. In that sense, man is greater than a god, potentially.

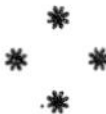

It depends upon how you look at it; the movement is the same. In the small speck the Vast wants to realise itself, even in this tiny speck. Sri Aurobindo observes somewhere that the Divine is as much present in the huge as in the microscopic. The pressure of consciousness is the same, the quality of consciousness is the same. It is only the illusion of quantity. The Divine in his vast wanted to translate himself into the microscopic. The Divine in his infinity wanted to indwell and manifest in the most fragmented finiteness. It is a totally different condition from a natural infinitude.

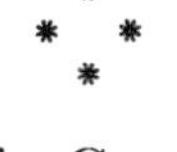

The Comet

It's like a double-edged knife; it cuts both ways. It is significant, that is true. The last time when a comet came — in 1960 or 1961, Mother spoke of a golden being whom she met in the comet, who had brought a special substance to be spread all over the earth. It was the golden substance of the Supramental world, she said. Now when the present comet came a number of people had predicted that spiritually it was not a good sign, that we would be in for a difficult dark period in the spiritual life of humanity. I came to know that a few days before the seventeenth of November when the attention of a holy man was drawn to the comet, he said that some great spiritual personality was about to pass away. That person did not know anything about our Ashram or Mother. After the seventeenth, when again that person was met, and when the tail of the comet was clearly visible, he said that the person had left. So there can't be a general rule as to whether these comets are indicative of good or bad; we can take it that they are indicative of certain significant movements. But usually in Indian astrology these comets are not very much welcomed.

Would you say then, the comet signifies a strong change?

Some change. It may be for the good, it may be for the bad. It all depends — even a bad thing ultimately does something good, doesn't it? It depends upon how we look at it, and with what perspective we look. I believe they're talking of a new comet at present? Perhaps it will now do good.

23

Samadhi

When I was a small boy, I was fond of reading stories. I remember reading of a princess who, while hunting in the forest with her retinue, came across an anthill with two bright shining spots. She was intrigued by them and wondered what they were. She took a sharp grass blade and pierced the sparkling holes. Immediately there was a flow of blood and the pretty princess was bewildered. Her followers rushed forward and it was discovered that what she had thought to be an anthill was in fact a sage who had been meditating for a long time. Ants had built a hill around his body which was immobile and what she had taken to be sparkling dots were his eyes. That the sage, in keeping with the traditions of the times, cursed the princess and that it took a lot of bother and trouble to get out of the curse is another story which need not concern us today.

I enjoyed it as a story and considered it as a poetical imagination. I left it there. Years later, when I was studying history in a higher secondary school, I read that when the British first came to India and, as a measure of consolidating their power in the country, started laying down railroads which necessitated the digging of the earth for hundreds of miles, they came across human figures in a sitting position. They were not dead, but obviously buried there. I recalled the anthill incident and it amazed me to know that men could live for hundreds of years in a particular state. I was told they were historical records; and particularly during the days of the Indian mutiny in 1857, a number of such discoveries were recorded.

There have been reports in recent times of saints, sages,

found sitting in a still posture for months together without food, without water. Some of these yogis, eager to win applause, have given public performances. There were some as near as a hundred miles from Pondicherry, asking to be buried alive for ten days, twenty days or thirty days and issuing instructions how the closed pit was to be opened, how a little bit of butter or camphor was to be rubbed slowly in the center of their head by their disciples and how finally they were to be helped back into active consciousness. Government authorities, the police, doctors have all attended such functions and testified to the truth of the phenomena.

There is, about three or four hundred miles from Madras, a famous centre of spiritual potency where a spiritual leader with a large religious following decided to close his earthly career by being buried alive in a prepared tomb. So on the appointed day, he sat down, took up his posture in the tomb and went into deep meditation. Bricks were laid over the tomb and it was closed. He had told the people that though his physical ministry was over, his spiritual ministry would last for another three hundred years. It is in the government records that when, some fifty years or so later, the Government of Madras wanted to acquire the adjoining land, the people raised such an outcry that the Governor of the province visited that place to settle the matter. During his visit he saw in a dream a venerable figure walking out of the tomb, coming to him and telling him, "Yes, this land belongs to this temple, this monastery. Do not disturb it." The Governor dropped all proceedings, returned to his headquarters and had it recorded in the government papers that as a result of that dream encounter, he had decided to drop the proposal to acquire the lands.

Now there are a number of instances of what is called the phenomena of yogic trance, what we in Sanskrit and Sanskrit-derived languages call *samadhi*. It is a natural culmination of the yoga of knowledge, which we have been considering so long, to practise the indrawing of one's consciousness or awareness more and more, away from external preoccupations and converging one's faculties and consciousness to one objective, may be inward or upward. The purpose is to release the consciousness, to focus the consciousness on a point, on a level, deeper or higher, till it is completely lost to its surroundings. Necessarily, in that context, it means a withdrawal from the world and after all the aim of the traditional yoga of knowledge is to reject the world, if not as a falsehood, as an inferior order of reality.

Even in the traditional yoga of love, of devotion, this increasing concentration of consciousness inward, away from contact with the external things, is cultivated in order to prepare the soul to be entirely occupied with the object of its adoration, so that it may lose itself in the presence and be nothing more than a receptacle for the bliss that flows from the Divine. In any case, the human consciousness is withdrawn, directed elsewhere, away from the world.

Surely, this cannot be the role of trance in a yoga that we have been pursuing, the Integral yoga. Here one goes into the condition of trance not to draw away from the world, but to acquire a state of consciousness akin to the Divine Consciousness — the highest possible for the human system — and turn to the world from that poise, to think and to act in that newly acquired and acclimatised consciousness. What are these grades of consciousness that the mind has to traverse, that the mind has to tread? This is a legitimate question.

That what man is conscious of normally is only a fringe of his being, is a fact that is being increasingly discovered in modern psychology and parapsychology, but it is taken as an axiomatic truth in Indian psychology. He lives only fragmentarily. There are grades after grades, levels after levels of consciousness which loom over his little physical consciousness from all sides. There is behind his extrovert consciousness a large subliminal consciousness which extends itself into superconscient heights, and also goes down to the subconscient depths. There is, besides, the environmental consciousness, what we call the circumconscient, surrounding him. Of all the entire consciousness that is massed in and around man, he lives only on a little fragment.

The Indian psychologists speak of four states of consciousness: the waking state, the dream state, the sleep state and the transcendent. Corresponding to each level of consciousness, there is the waking Self, the dream Self, the sleep Self and the fourth, the supreme or the transcendent. All these, they take care to point out, are not four different persons, four different entities, but the one transcendent self that poises itself on these four levels to draw the experience of each level of existence. The range of each successive level is wider, larger than the previous one.

We understand very well that when we speak of the waking state it means a state of awareness in which we are conscious of all the external things, mostly through our senses or the sense-based mental operations. We also understand that when we speak of the dream state it means when we are withdrawn from active occupation with the outside world; we are turned inward and luxuriate in an unfettered movement of our subtler senses. The physical senses are asleep, but the subtler senses behind them are active. We expand, physical distances melt away, we enter into another order of existence where things are faster, where physical barriers break down. But all the while they have a resemblance to the state of things on the physical plane.

By the sleep state these psychologists of yoga mean a dreamless sleep, where is no movement of dream, only a blank. When we come out of it, we know we existed, but we can't say, we can't describe what happened. This is called *Sushupti*, deep, dreamless sleep. The self of this dreamless sleep state is the causal self, the self of the causal body. It is the gnostic self, this causal body in which the person exists in the deep sleep state, is the sheath of the gnostic soul. Beyond is the transcendent, the absolute.

When we speak of the sleep self, it is not right to understand it to mean "self that is asleep". In fact, they take care to use other adjectives, saying that he is *prajna*, the wise one, the luminous one, the Lord of Knowledge. He is wide awake, more awake than any of the selves below. But it is called "sleep" because that is the only word to denote an order of things of which our waking, or even our dream self cannot take cognisance.

It is possible to enter into trance on any of these levels. It is possible for a man to confine himself to the waking state and get into trance, get into samadhi, losing contact with all the rest but not going higher. This is a point that I want you to note. It is possible to go into samadhi on the dream level. It is also possible, though more difficult, to go into samadhi in the sushupti state. What happens when one practises this yoga of Patanjali or the Rajayoga as it is called, or the Hathayoga, which we will discuss in our next session, is that one is confined to the physical level. By concentration, by force of will, one withdraws the outgoing faculties, holds them together, and cultivates the habit of keeping them in one position. One need not believe in God, one need not want to reach God; it is a matter of existence, a matter of consciousness, awareness. Once one withdraws the various faculties of the consciousness inward, away from the external awareness, they get fixed.

Even, in that state when the whole thing is drawn and centred in one position, the whole of the breath gets centred there. It is an automatic and a spontaneous operation, that as the consciousness gets centered in a narrow and narrower place, the breath also narrows itself, and it holds. It is a yogic technique of joining the breath with the stream of consciousness, with the line of consciousness, and holding it. At that time all the physical operations of the body may be suspended, and for want of sustenance from the life-force which is indrawn with the consciousness, the heart-beats may appear to stop, the pulse may appear to stop. There may be no movement, and as there is no movement, no wear and tear of the body; life continues in its subtle form, in its narrowed circle within. Outwardly, the person is dead. No food is necessary, no air is necessary because in that state one does not need to breathe in the normal way to live; life exists by itself. There is no interchange; one is as in a sealed chamber. This, then, is the condition; one need not be spiritual, one need not believe in the Divine. It is a matter of technique, practice and endurance. It is a *siddhi*, an accomplishment that is aimed at in Hathayoga where the technique is only of *asanas* to accustom the body to certain irregular states, *pranayama*, the regulation and control of breath to bring it into a desired movement, functioning.

This would explain to you the phenomenon of which you may be reading in journals and papers of yogis living for hundreds of years, lost in their trance, meditation. It is a *siddhi* which, however, has no significance from the point of view of spiritual evolution. It has no meaning for humanity. How does it help? If I acquire a higher state of consciousness and use it to shut myself in, to live long, to be away from all circumstances of life, how does it help the rest? It is an individual *siddhi* which is depreciated in the higher yogic tradition.

There is then, going into trance on the dream level. One does not actually sleep, but when one withdraws from the physical state, the next stage is where the subtler being, the subtler levels of consciousness unfold themselves, the subtler senses begin to operate. If one chooses, one can become aware even of the physical universe around through the subtler senses. One can hear, one can even see through the subtle eye what is going on. One becomes aware of grades of existence which are larger and higher than the physical. Various planes reveal their contents and if one is so minded, one goes to explore them, or one shuts one's eye to them. It is to be noted that the condition of a physical dream and the condition of a trance-dream are totally different from each other. In the normal dream that we have in the normal state of sleep, it is all a jumble of delayed reactions to touches and impacts of the day-to-day life, reactions of the senses — which are half-aware or three-quarters awake — to impacts from outside, imaginations, subconscious impressions, all these coming up together. This is what happens, an unregulated, confusing movement which tires. Of course there are types of dreams which are premonitory dreams which are pleasant, but normally, for a man in ignorance, this is the state of dreams.

In the trance dream, however, there is a complete regulation of the government of the subtle senses — regulated imaginations, regulated perceptions. One sees, one gets the thoughts, one hears the sounds, but all in a regulated and controlled manner. It is here, in the course of becoming conscious of levels of life which are higher than the physical, that one comes across, and if one chooses, one can take cognisance of what is called the subtle, etheric atmosphere where all that has happened, all that is happening and all that is to happen are found recorded. This is a continuous process that goes on in the universe, but the contents of the subtle etheric state are shut in due to the gross sediments or layers of the physical ether. In the dream state of trance the eye is opened to what is recorded on that film of subtle ether, which is called in Sanskrit *Chit-Akash*, the sky of consciousness.

Sri Aurobindo describes graphically how what is recorded concerns not only the past, not only the present, but even the future; it is the memory of the future. How does the memory of the future come? He answers that to the eye of knowledge, the past, present and the future are all mapped out. It takes time for things to precipitate on earth, but on that level they are all laid out. If one has eyes to see, the perception to catch, one can know anything. It is a ray of this knowledge that comes in our waking states now and then. We call it clairaudience, clairvoyance.

After this state of dream level the yogin withdraws still inwards and there he enters into a state of which he can only report, "I was. I was in a state of bliss, but I do not know for what". This is because the human apparatus of recording as it is is not yet equipped, is not yet developed enough to keep the memory, to elongate the knowledge of the contents of that consciousness in the waking state. This is the status of the gnostic self in dreamless sleep, dreamless state.

Still deeper, one becomes aware of the self of bliss, where even in that trance state one is flooded with bliss. You may ask, is that all? No, above the bliss-self, beyond it is the self of pure, sheer existence. Even the word "bliss" does not do justice to that state, where bliss is only one of the vibrations. It is a state of pure existence, it is a state of the Absolute.

It is difficult for man to connect his waking state with all these states of trance. But by practice, in the measure in which the psychic being opens and learns to grow into the deeper and higher states of consciousness and hold the contents of that consciousness in its state, it is possible to forge a bridge between the outer states of consciousness and the deeper and still deeper states of trance. These states of trance do not have the same significance, the same role to play in the Integral Yoga as they have in the traditional yogas. They are meant to connect the waking consciousness to the different and higher levels of existence, normalise those states through peak periods of meditations called trance, establish links between the different levels of consciousness so that all those levels of consciousness which are realised could be gradually and increasingly embodied in the waking condition and utilised to manifest the Divine who embodies himself in these several states of consciousness.

One can arrive at these states of consciousness without going into trance by opening oneself, keeping oneself receptive to the descents of the higher states of consciousness, keeping always linked to the external life. Without getting lost into the depths of trance, it is possible to receive in oneself first the reflections, then by identity the very body of these states of higher consciousness and normalise them in oneself so that in due time one can function simultaneously on so many levels of consciousness. All the three or four selves can operate in the integral man, for after all, that is the significance of the *integral* man.

Questions

In the formative stages of the psychic being being developed and brought forth, how does what you have said relate to its coming forward. Does it come forward first and then make these bridges, or do the bridges encourage the psychic being to come forward?

As the psychic being forms itself and takes possession of the being, more and more, it grows in stature, and in the very growth of this stature points of contact are established with higher levels of consciousness and it is through these points of contact that the higher levels of consciousness get entry into the waking condition of the seeker. One does not have to make a conscious effort as in the traditional yogic trance, but one has to keep vigilant and expand oneself according to the demands of the psychic being. As the consciousness grows, one has to cooperate in the expansion of the rule of the psychic being.

In this yoga it is a speciality that once the psychic being is awake, that takes charge of the sadhana and the tact lies in attuning oneself, the rest of one's nature, to the awakened psychic being. The psychic, after all, is a spark of God, of the Divine, and as it awakes it links the individual to the Divine above or behind. The psychic being, you may say, forges the links by itself.

In reference to these Akashic records, are there occult lines that one sees or are there also possibilities that one sees?

What are normally called Akashic records in the Theosophical and allied literature are supposed transcripts on the vital levels, on the surfaces of the subtle existence. They are not the true records of the Chit-Akash. These are scripts on subtle-physical or vital levels which may misguide. They are not of Truth origin.

It was only two days ago that I had to go through a book called the *Aquarian Gospel of Jesus Christ*. The whole book of two hundred pages is compiled from Akashic records by someone in America, between four and six in the morning — that is supposed to be the best period to understand these things. He worked for over six months. All kinds of details are there; Christ is supposed to have spent eighteen years in India, Tibet, Orissa, Kashmir. Dialogues are recorded. The dialogues are quite interesting but certainly they can't be authentic. They lack that ring. They are dramatic enough, interesting, as you read and enjoy them, but they don't have those vibrations. The thing is, they are not the purer strata of cosmic consciousness on which the records are placed or things get recorded, but interferences on the intermediate levels by entities which amuse themselves. There is a realm where possibilities abound. There is a realm where what is certain, determined, is clear. One must develop the discrimination to distinguish.

It is not very comforting to know that ninety percent of our life, spiritual or material, is in the realm of possibilities. That the thing is going to manifest, that we are going to realise, is a certainty. But the time factor is in the realm of possibilities. Whether I realise God in my present life, or in another life, is in the realm of possibilities. The certainty is that once I have set on the path, I am going to realise it because unless I was ready for it, unless I was meant for it, I would not have been put on the path.

I have a question regarding inventions. Copyrights for inventions often appear at the same time but in areas quite distant from each other. Is it possible for one to go into these realms and become aware of some invention that is not yet manifest?

Yes. Theoretically it is possible because all that we invent here is there pre-arranged on a higher plane. What happens normally is that when that formation descends into the earth atmosphere, whoever is open to it, in whichever country, receives it and he expresses it in the language that is natural to him, in the way that is normal to him. That is how you will find the same inventions or the same ideas have been expressed or brought into existence in different countries at the same time. It is possible for one to go in consciousness to those levels, seize those things, and if one is developed, to bring it consciously and embody it on earth. It is possible.

But normally a person who has that developed consciousness to be able to do it, does not do it because he knows that the earth conditions are not yet ready for that formation to take birth here, because when the conditions are ready it descends by itself if it is intended to form a part of the manifestation.

Leonardo da Vinci: There was an effort from his end which stimulated those higher formations, designs etc. to precipitate themselves. Largely, they come from above, but he was ready. His mind had formed the grooves into which the things could flow. In fact he was a being who was projected on earth precisely to precipitate those formations in earth existence. He was not an evolutionary being like others. He was what is called a *vibhuti*, an emanation.

From what plane was he a projection or an emanation?

From the typal plane of those things which he brought out. There is a typal world of art, of music, typal world of these scientific things where they are preenvisaged and sorted out. They can be anywhere between the subtle physical and the mental. These are all parts of the manifested universe.

Before they are manifested on the physical plane, they are all marshalled and kept ready on those higher planes. Certain musicians are emanations from the music world may be vital, subtle physical, I can't say. But certainly it is not what some think, that they are from a divine plane or a truth plane. They belong to certain intermediate planes of existence where the movements of art, music and the like have been in a state of certain perfection. In Indian scriptures we call these the world of Gandharvas. They are the gods of harmony, beauty, music. There is a vital world of beauty, there is a vital world of music — it can move masses, it can inspire one, the right way or the wrong way. There is a vital world of poetry just as there is a mental world of poetry.

If a collective group of artists wanted to draw down the highest possible consciousness, would there be a way to work towards that?

Yes. If one aspires to the Truth, the Highest Divine that one has got fixed in his aspiration, to reveal itself in the appropriate or the highest art forms that are to manifest the truth, that truth chooses forms from the art world and precipitates them. Whether we receive them without deforming them is another question. Usually our own ideas, our own formations interfere — if they are not my own or your own then the collective ideas. Between that world and our physical world there are other beings; they also may interfere, dilute. So there are so many intervening possibilities between the release of the right form from that plane and the reception of them here on earth. But it is possible to move the highest to reveal the right forms of art, of music, or architecture which can render the highest truth to man. That is possible.

In the course of creation, perfect worlds are formed, what Sri Aurobindo calls the typal worlds — where art is raised to its highest potency, music is developed to its highest. They form the stuff, the substance for the creative spirit to work with. If the power that comes in answer to our aspiration is from the Truth plane, the stuff that is chosen and precipitated on earth will be imbued with that Truth. If we are content to receive guidance from an intermediate power which pleases us or our sense of aesthesis, it will be that order of art creation.

The Mother's personality continues, but not in the sense of a physical personality.* Personality need not be always physical. The physical is a front; behind the physical there are so many other personalities, so there is a personality that continues to preside and hide, and it is very concrete. It may not be physical, it may not be physically perceptible, but it is there in the subtle form. The personality continues. Things are not dissolved into an impersonality. Even when she was here in the body, she had both. Sri Aurobindo had explained in a different context though that as a personality she channeled the grace. You can receive grace by approaching her in her personal form. But in her impersonal form in her impersonal way, she is the universal power, the consciousness which works according to the laws of the universe. So she has simultaneously two levels of functioning, the personal and the impersonal. Her leaving the physical body does not make a difference to this truth of her manifestation. She is, and she will continue to be, a personalised divinity for the work that she has undertaken.

How should we approach the Mother now?

Each one will see her in the form that is familiar to him or in which he conceives of the Mother. The same embodiment reveals itself to the perceiving eye according to its previous formation. To those who have seen Mother physically, she will reveal herself in that form — may be with a different luminosity and others, but essentially it will be in the same form.

* The Mother left her physical body on November 17, 1973

24

Hathayoga

This time we could as well start with a story, albeit a real one. Some two or three years ago there was a sensation in the Western part of India when one of the holy men who performs miracles such as producing ashes, fountain pens, wrist watches and the like by the sheer wave of his hand, was given a challenge by one who called himself a yogi. The latter said, "If this holy person has real occult powers let him repeat a feat that I am going to perform. The feat that I propose to do in full view of the public is to walk on water. If this gentleman also can do that, then and then only shall I admit his spiritual attainments."

Well, to prove his own credentials, he was asked to demonstrate his powers first. A number of newspapers and journals in Bombay took up his cause and a heavy-pressured news propaganda was let loose. Hundreds of people from outside the city poured into Bombay. The whole city was littered with placards, editorials were written in papers, guides were posted, and it was like a carnival where thousands of people were gathered. Suitable arrangements had been made, tickets were naturally issued, and a lot of money was collected. More than Indian newsmen, American newsmen who were in India at that time rushed to Bombay with their cameras and movies. And I must confess that in my corner of the country I was also a bit excited and was following the event in the newspapers.

When I looked for the bold headline in the papers the next morning, I was disappointed that there was none. But in the corner of a middle page there was an item mentioning that the huge crowd that had gathered for the demonstration had been disappointed because the said yogi, although he did come to show his power, when he stepped into the water and was about to take next step, fell into the water. The disappointment was acute because it was known that he had been showing this feat in private gatherings. This was the first time in public, but a number of friends and some experts had testified to having seen him demonstrate this power. Later when the newsmen plagued him and asked him why he had failed, the yogi's explanation was interesting. He had been told that some people said that he had failed because of the curses of the other holy man, whom he had had the temerity to challenge. He dismissed this reason and said, "I don't know if you will believe me. What happened was that unexpectedly I developed a cold, but matters had gone too far and the function had to be held. I had hoped to control the nasal cold, but I could not, with the result that the particular poise in the body which had to be taken by a special process of breathing, pranayam, could not be taken as the nose was blocked." So that was why he could not make the body lighter than water and failed. There were reports that he tried thereafter when he was in good health, to repeat the experiment, but I suppose the nervous shock that he had had at that time proved to be an insurmountable psychological barrier against any future success.

I have brought this incident to your notice to underline the principles of Hathayoga, which is the theme of our talk today. We have seen that the high aim of the traditional yoga of knowledge is to go into samadhi, a state which is much more than what is called in the West trance. It is a concentrated state of consciousness, awareness when the mind is completely lost to anything else except the object on which it is dwelling, a further state of samadhi being the complete identification of the consciousness with the object. There is no more concentrating on the object for the consciousness is lost in the object.

The aim of the traditional yoga of knowledge is to lose oneself in the Reality, in the consciousness of Brahman, in which there is nothing else but the One. This state of samadhi is the object, in some way or other, of the many lines of yoga that have been prevalent in India. One of the main yogas is the Hathayoga, the yoga that concentrates on the physical body.

The yoga of knowledge concerns itself with the development of mind and the mental faculties; the yoga of love with the heart, the emotional being, the evocation of the psychic; the yoga of works with the dynamisation of the will of man for the attainment of the divine Consciousness; while Hathayoga aims at striking a balance and a relation between the body and the soul in such a way that the soul can move, can function as freely in the physical body as it does at present in its subtle, causal body.

The normal human body of which most of us are aware is only a vehicle, an inert, mechanical dull vehicle for the life-energy that circulates in it. It obstructs every upward movement, every forward movement of the life-force or the mind-energy that circulates in it. The Hathayogin seeks to so produce and develop the body that instead of being a hindrance to the free movements of the mind and life energies, it will support them, give them its strength, and itself develop into a direct vehicle of God.

The process of Hathayoga is first a system of postures, what are called *asanas*, physical postures. Now asana does not mean only a physical posture. Originally an asana meant that poise, whether physical or mental, spiritual or psychological, in which one is most at ease and in tune with something deeper or higher that one seeks. Such a poise is an asana that is most conducive to one's development and progress. In a limited context, an asana is a particular physical posture which sets the body in a position in which it can stay undisturbed for as long as one wants. Normally we find that it is impossible for us to sit in one stationary poise. We tend to move, if not the whole body at least some part of it. When we sit for a while, there is an accumulation of the life-force; either it has to be worked out, or it has to be spilled. In either case as the life-force accumulates, as the mind begins to think, in the body there is a certain restlessness; the body cannot contain the force. It begins to sway, move from side to side.

Hathayoga has worked out a number of physical postures, some complicated, some simple, by which, apart from the toning up of the physical body and the strengthening of the muscles, it puts the whole system into a kind of immobility in which the physical body forgets itself and acts as an unmoving pedestal for whatever use one chooses to make of it. There are as many as eighty-four asanas or postures, though only about sixteen or so are considered to be the main ones, the rest being permutations and combinations of the latter. Each asana has its own steps, and the precise benefits from each asana are recorded. For our purpose it is enough if the body is accustomed to periods of immobile unmoving postures. Secondly, it must be developed in such a way that it can contain any amount of life-force or the life energy that is either invited into it or that pours into it from the universal store of life energy. In the beginning, as the energy pours in, there is a shaking of the body but these asanas in which the body is trained to sit for a while in a concentrated manner accustom the body not only to bear the inrush of energy, but develop the capacity to increasingly hold more and more of the supply of life energy.

Along with the asanas there comes as the next step, *pranayama*. Pranayama is the name given to a series of exercises that aim to regulate, arrest and prolong the span of the life movement, the movement of the life-force in the body. As you are aware, the life-force has a number of functions. The first function, breathing, is the key to the other four movements. There is the "breath of life", as they say, breathing in, then comes the expelling of the air that is breathed in, then there is the operation of equalisation between the in-breathing and the out-breathing, then there is the spreading of the life breath that is taken in equally in all the parts, then there is the operation of exit through the head. The life-force is ejected through the head at the time of the parting from the body.

These are the five main operations of the life-force. There are five other subsidiary operations into which we need not now enter. Now, breathing — the main and the first operation — holds the key to the rest. By first equalising the period of inspiration and expiration, a certain rhythm is arrived at. With this established rhythm, there is an automatic improvement in the flow of thoughts, because the mind and the life are intimately connected. If you observe yourself closely you will find that when you are excited, when the thinking rushes in a fury, the whole of the life-force, the breathing is restless. You breathe fast, you breathe hard. Similarly, when you are lost in concentration, in contemplation, in meditation, you will see the breathing slowing down. The reverse can also be true. If by any kind of process of control you slow down the breathing, it has an immediate and a direct effect on the movement of the thoughts. That is why pranayama has been given so much importance in traditional yogas. We hear people always complaining that when they close their eyes for meditation there is a rush of thoughts, the mind runs in a hundred directions. They ask how to control the mind. The ancients offered this solution. They asked you to regulate your breathing; to begin with equalising the period of inbreathing and outbreathing.

In one of his lectures in the West, Swami Vivekananda gave a simple exercise to the seekers. He said: place your finger on one nostril and breathe in deeply through the other. Don't hold it, but immediately with the same speed, let it out through the other nostril. Then through the same nostril breathe in and again with the same speed let it out through the other. Do ten times this way and ten times the other. You may do it at any time and you will see the result immediately. There is a certain calming of the system; the mind breathes easy.

This is the simplest exercise. Then at a later stage comes a period of holding the breath that you breathe in. You hold it for some time and then let it out. More attention is to be paid to the act of breathing out than breathing in because one always tends to do that faster. Breathing out has to be controlled, it has to be slowed down. The whole principle is to bring the process of breathing, the process of the working of the life-force, under one's control.

With this the first step in the purification of the system is effected. For regular, disciplined exercises in the regulation of life energies result not only in the quieting of the mind, but in the opening up of the clogged cells of the nervous system. All over the nervous system there are areas which are clogged, not so much physically as psycho-physically. Emotions, desires, past associations, physical habits, all these clog the movement of the life-force and it is normally unable to circulate in the whole nervous system in a healthy way. That is why there are imbalances in the system which when they accumulate, express themselves as physical illnesses. This system of the regulation of breathing, the regulation of the life-force, the breath of life, aims at opening up all the channels of the nervous system and assuring a smooth flow of the energies, not only the physical energies but the life energies, the mental energies, psychic energies and the spiritual energies. When all these are left to flow without interruption, the whole system gets toned up.

Afterwards, once the system is purified, there is the next step of concentration. All the energies at every level are more easily assembled, marshalled together and poured on the object of pursuit. Whether it is meditation, or worship or thinking, whatever the activity, all the energies in the system are assembled without difficulty and raised to their maximum potential.

Third comes liberation. After purification of the system, after concentration and the galvanising of the diverse energies and the monitoring of them to the purpose in view, the third step is liberation, the liberation of the inner being from its clampings to outer nature and the release, either in the inward or the upward direction as chosen.

These are the three main steps of Hathayoga. At this stage, Hathayoga develops into Rajayoga, and Rajayoga is essentially a more psycho-physical system than Hathayoga, which emphasises more the physical, the material aspect of the situation. One inevitable result of these asanas, of the bringing the body functions completely under control, of the developing the body potentiality to its maximum and thus acquiring control of the life-force, the breathing, is that not only is there a change in the balancing of the different operations in the system, but also a changing of the balance between the forces outside and those inside.

For instance, as one develops in this line, the force of the earth's gravitation on the physical body is lessened. One can, if one chooses, get lighter than the earth, lighter than air, lighter than water. All of you, who have read the biography of Sri Aurobindo, know how in the Alipore jail people saw Sri Aurobindo sitting in meditation about a foot above the ground. And when he was asked about it, he said he was not conscious of it, he had not done it deliberately. He was doing pranayama at that time, the balance had been altered and the body getting lighter, just floated up. Normally Hathayogins live very much on the physical surface, but Sri Aurobindo, as you know, was always concentrated within, so he was not aware of this physical manifestation of levitation. People can make their bodies heavier also so that they can't be moved, can't be lifted. It is possible, by certain siddhis or achievements in hathayoga or rajayoga to acquire the powers of reducing the body form to a microscopic size, of magnifying to a huge size, and many other feats. These are the wonders that attract so many vulgar minds to yoga and serve to debase the whole system. Such people lose sight of the lofty ideals with which they started. And that is why the ancients severely discouraged the pursuit of these achievements. For though there is nothing unspiritual about them, they distract the consciousness, if one is not vigilant, from the central pursuit.

After the body is accustomed to sit for long periods of immobility without getting restless, it is also a part of this system, with the aid of other processes, to which we shall come in our next talk, to awaken the potent serpent power at the base of the spine and lead it up through the spinal column from centre to centre until it reaches its highest peak over the head in the thousand-petaled lotus. It is understood that neither this serpent power, nor these centres, which are called *chakras* or wheels, are located in the physical body.

You may have heard of the Italian surgeon who operated upon a dead body and challenged people to show him the centres and the serpent power. Well, all yogas, all occult sciences are one in maintaining that these centres are not precisely the ganglionic centres which medical science is familiar with. They are centres in the subtle body which have corresponding effects in the physical body. Those centres in the subtle body correspond to certain areas in the physical body. That is why when these centres are awake, one feels their action in the physical body and one tends to believe that they are centred in the physical body.

Questions

What would be the length of time that one in our yoga might spend each day over one certain asana?

Well, Sri Aurobindo has said that these laborious and difficult processes of Hathayoga and Rajayoga are not built into this system of Integral Yoga, though their aims have been kept in view. But they can be made use of in the preliminary stages, or up to any stage as long as they are useful.

Personally, after having been here for quite some time, having known something of this yoga, having known also from my personal experience, the difficulties of hundreds of sadhaks and seekers with whom I had occasion to talk, after reading thousands of letters from all over the world, I feel that some acquaintance with the simpler asanas and the simpler processes of regulation of breath is necessary to give a good, stable grounding to the seeker.

The Upanishads are one in saying that the posture has to be erect. They say that the chest, the nose and the neck are to be in a straight position. It is most important that the spine should be erect. Look at a person who does asanas; you will never find him stooping. He will always sit erect, whether he reads, whether he takes food, whether he sits on the beach and watches the sea, he will always sit erect. And that assures that the breathing goes on in its full span. If, at that time, there is a descent or an ascent it will not be hindered by the posture. And, also, if we sit normally for about half an hour or forty-five minutes, we tend to move our legs, our heads. That is a certain distraction, a minus factor.

We must familiarise ourselves, practise some of these preliminary asanas and postures in order to make the physical basis strong enough to stand periods of meditation or concentration. We must keep ourselves open and unhindered physically to the downflow and the action of the yoga force from whatever plane it comes.

Similarly with breathing. Breathing exercises reduce, during meditation, the difficulty of distraction by thoughts at least by fifty percent. I am not going to start an ashram at any time, but if anyone who wants to start one were to consult me,

I would advise him to introduce these simple exercises in asanas and pranayam.

Have you seen a person who practises *pranayama*? He may not be highly spiritual but there is a certain glow on the face, there is a certain contentment — may be a superficial contentment but contentment all the same — in his being.

If along with the physical culture and the gymnastic exercises, some attention is paid to this side of the yogic science, the results would be much better. One has to utilise them but one cannot be imprisoned by these processes.

With certain exaggerations which are very natural to the human mind in ignorance, one tends to look upon the asanas and the pranayama as sufficient in themselves. It must always be remembered that an asana is a means, pranayama is a means, even as meditation is a means. Meditation is not an end in itself; meditation is important, concentration is important, because they can bring about certain states of consciousness which are favourable to the reception of higher vibrations, we begin to tune ourselves to the higher, diviner consciousness.

So my answer is: it depends upon each person as to how much attention he gives to this preliminary but important aspect of the matter. This preliminary precaution, if taken in time, reduces the labour of yoga.

Is it possible, since we are interested not only in the Integral Yoga, but in the yoga of transformation when "Even the cells shall remember God" that research in Hathayoga can be directed towards transformation?

Hathayoga provides the essential field of all the lines of yoga for experimental research. And most of the research that is at present being conducted by American scientists in India is in the fields of Hathayoga and Rajayoga. Because they lend themselves to be measured on the physical plane, these changes of vibrations, changes of circulation and the speed of certain things can be recorded by the machines. So a lot of research has been done as to which asana leads to which results, demonstrable results.

If you read *Light of Yoga* by Iyengar you will find that he has developed this science of Hathayoga and Rajayoga in terms of modern thought. You will see all the data have been recorded in a scientific manner. How the pulse rate slows down, how the breathing changes, and then I.Q.S. and all those things have been recorded. I have no interest in them. But changes in states of consciousness, the quality of consciousness, can't be registered by physical machines. You will have to evolve a more subtle instrument. I can understand the state of your consciousness only if I have a consciousness that can connect itself with it. When I develop my consciousness into an instrument to receive impacts and relay them to my perceiving intelligence, that will be the machine as far as consciousness is concerned. But the rest of it, the less subtle part of the matter can be researched. But here, when it is a matter of consciousness, what in Indian systems we call the authentic word of experience, you can't insist upon a physical proof.

Indian science speaks of four kinds of knowledge. One is empirical knowledge; you experiment, you see the results and fortify that knowledge. There is next knowledge by inference; you observe something a hundred times and then you say that when this happens the cause must be this. Then there is the knowledge of authentic experience; when a person has had a profound experience, his word carries conviction. When you don't have the experience, and if you find that he is otherwise honest, straightforward, truthful, when he speaks of something which you have not experienced, it stands to reason that you accept his word. How many of us have experienced the supramental or the overmental consciousness? Why do we accept Mother's and Sri Aurobindo's word in these matters? It is convincing, it carries conviction. Their very words are loaded with experience, they come like bullets and you feel it can't be otherwise. You can't do research into that with the present instruments. When you evolve different instruments you can. Each order of reality has its own means of verification.

(Concerning guidelines for dealing with someone who is angry)

The Mother said that on such occasions you must stay absolutely quiet, without participating in the movement of anger on the part of the other. At that time you have to be quiet. Think of peace, call in peace, let him spend himself out. But if you were to contradict, if you were to point out that he is unreasonable, you participate in his movement of anger and it thrives. You have to, literally, close yourself; then even if the impact takes place, it is on the superficial layers, and it just dies out. As in many other things you have to be conscious. If you are conscious, there is an automatic bolting the door; you don't let it in. Movements of anger, movements of envy, movements of passion, all strike, but if you are cool, quiet, they cannot enter. If you are nervous, if you react, they can. You must learn not to react in any way.

. . . *If you try to keep this attitude, you make them even more angry.*

The right attitude for a spiritual person, if one has provoked another person by one's own failure, is to admit it immediately, and the anger dies down. One has to admit honestly "I am sorry, I have done it.". The thunder is over. He may go on shouting for some time, but he loses the impetus. But if one is angry, without justification — really there can't be justification for anger — then, the Mother said humorously, take a cup of water and give it to him first. And tell him that you will talk after he finishes drinking that glass of water. By the time he finishes, his anger would have gone down.

(Referring to the position of the hands in meditation)

Meditation in our yoga is not done only while sitting. One can meditate when one walks, one can meditate when one runs, one can meditate when one stands. Meditation becomes a sort of concurrent process as one develops. So, in the very nature of things, there can't be a fixed position of the hands. Though in the ancient texts it is mentioned that some positions of the hands conduce a favourable movement in the system. For those who find it necessary, they can be utilised. They are called *mudras*, the placing of fingers in certain ways. They attract certain occult movements and they contribute favourably.

These are all part of rituals; usually they observe these things during worship. They may have been necessary at a certain stage in the development of the human mind, the human emotions, but today, psychologically man has developed so much that these outer means of ritual, elaborate postures, are not so indispensable.

Normally Mother would not give much importance to these things. She always laid stress on development of consciousness, the right attitude, vigilance; she always laid stress on the psychological side. But all of a sudden I have seen Mother saying that for this purpose the asanas are good, for that purpose pranayam is good. I have seen Mother recognising their role in particular situations, though, as a rule, she was not minded to give them importance in her scheme of things.

But she was aware of the whole system, and I remember on one occasion when Madam David-Neel, Mother's friend in the early days, wrote to her from France asking what was the position of *pranayama* in our yoga, Mother called three or four of us and asked us to give notes on *pranayama* and its use from our standpoint. I didn't write anything of my own at that time; I gave excerpts from Sri Aurobindo's writings in *The Synthesis* and she was very much satisfied. Her attitude in such matters was, "If that is your cup of tea, you have it."

In some of the Mother's writings, she has described how you have a dialogue with the vital or various parts of the being. And in

Hathayoga, from what I have seen, that kind of dialogue is carried on with physical parts. This dialogue with various parts of one's being, could this be carried further?

I suppose it is what we call in modern terms auto-suggestion. You go on saying to yourself what you should and what you should not be. You separate yourself from the body, from the vital, from the mental, you take your position as the *purusha*, and then you go on putting suggestions and your will. It is easier to do it that way than when you are identified with these parts. So they speak of separating oneself from nature and then educating the various parts of nature to fall in line. I believe that they have developed these things in very minute detail in the Buddhist systems.

Sri Aurobindo says that healing can be done through Hathayoga.

In the sense that the energies are directed in the place you want. Normally a system gets ill in a particular part either due to faulty functioning or inadequate supply of life-force there. By these exercises it is possible to become conscious of those parts and direct the stream of life energy in those areas. To that extent it is possible but I believe that there are also processes for reversing or modifying the flow of blood or the flow of energies. They are all intricate processes and they take the help of the Ayurveda, the Indian system of medicine from roots, leaves and herbs. They utilise it as a subsidiary help.

These advanced processes of Hathayoga take a lot of time, consume a lot of energy and they leave little time for anything else. Modern science has developed various ways of effecting cures rapidly, in a microscopic amount of time and it is wiser to take advantage of modern science where it is not harmful to the system and devote the time so gained to higher pursuits instead of being always preoccupied with the body, its illnesses and indispositions.

There should be a sense of proportion. I must ask myself whether the amount of energy and time I spend is worth spending in an overall perspective, on what I am doing. That perspective, the central purpose should never be lost sight of. It is a characteristic contribution of Sri Aurobindo and the Mother to look at things in their totality, to have a global view of things.

25

Rajayoga

We spoke last time of Hathayoga, which emphasises the physical body and the life force. We concluded on the note that at its best Hathayoga opens the door to Rajayoga — the yoga of the mind, which lays more emphasis upon the mind than upon either the life or the body. We must remember, however, that the mind depends for its functioning a good deal upon the life-force that is involved in the body. Modern science would have it that the birth is only of the physical body that is activated by the life energies and that neither the mind nor the soul have any independent existence. Some would go so far as to say that the mind and the soul are the epiphenomena of matter. They do not explain the many things that happen independent of the body and the life-force in the activities of the mind. But the ancient psycho-physical science of yoga in India has resolved this question of the dependence, and also the independence, of the mind as far as its relations with the life-force and the physical body are concerned. For yogic science recognises that behind the exterior physical body of which we are conscious and which we see, there is a subtle-physical body, what they call the life-body with which the soul is clothed when it sheds the physical body.

Now this subtle-physical body has got its own life-force and its own subtle substance. The subtle life-force that courses through the subtle physical body runs through a number of centres of concentration of energy — what are picturesquely called the lotuses — and from the bottom of the subtle physical body, crossing through these various centres, which represent, so to say, the convolutions of the subtle energy, the subtle life-force shoots up to the highest centre near the head, the seat of the superconscient consciousness.

This system of lotuses, or wheels as they are called, is almost exactly reproduced in the physical body along the spine in the several ganglionic centres. But remember that these lotuses of subtle energy are not situated in the physical body; they are not attached to the physical spinal column, they really exist in the subtle body and only their action impinges upon the corresponding areas along the spinal column of the physical body.

It is the aim of these yogic systems to arouse this primal energy in the subtle physical body by exerting pressure upon it, and this pressure is most easily exerted by joining the higher breath and the lower breath. When this pressure is exerted with concentration for a certain amount of time, the involved energy, the primal "energy", which is likened to a serpent coiled round itself three and a half times, is struck on its hood, as it were, and it rises up, opening in the process so to say windows on the several planes of existence which are connected with each centre, till the force rises to near the crown of the head, where there is what is called the superconscient Self, the Divine Self. And with this joining of the force from the lowest centre to the highest, there issues a shower of bliss and also a merger of the individual human consciousness with the Divine Consciousness which has its centre there. Naturally, this is an experience which needs to be repeated again and again before it organises itself in the system and develops into a permanent realisation. There is a regular science on the subject which is called the science of the Kundalini Yoga and in it, you will be interested to know, the several lotuses are so called because to the subtle vision the configurations of the subtle nerves look like so many petals of a lotus. The petals have been actually numbered beginning with four petals in the lotus at the base of the spine to six, eight, twelve, sixteen, two and finally a thousand — thousand represents a full, plenary figure, not necessarily a numerical thousand. And each one of these lotuses is pictured as hanging with its face down. As the force strikes them the lotuses turn upward and they remain that way; it represents the opening of the consciousness at that level. So each lotus blossoms till the force reaches the top, and when it comes down, lotus by lotus, they again turn downwards and close up. In the normal human system, only a fraction of this subtle pranic force is active — only as much as is necessary to sustain the normal life operations. It is only by yoga that a deeper potential is tapped and various forces are released which break the walls of the limiting physical organisation. And the regulation of breath, the elongation of breath — what we call pranayama — is the main means adopted in Rajayoga towards this end, but it is not the sole means.

As help to this exercise of the breath, there is the use of the mantra, the seed syllable, the potent syllable, which is repeated along with the breathing. This evokes certain spiritual vibrations and adds to the effort — adding a spiritual dimension to what would otherwise be a pure psycho-physical process; for a mantra is the sound-body of a divine entity. Each divine reality has its own sound form, and each mantra is revered as the sound-body of that deity. For particular ends, there are particular mantras, and it is laid down that whatever the purpose the first essential condition is to tap and release into operation, the hidden potential.

Sri Aurobindo has given a beautiful and graphic description of the process in his epic *Savitri*. Most of you have read *Savitri*. You remember the scene where, as the day of Satyavan's death draws near, Savitri spends her nights praying to the divine puissance, the Divine Mother. And one day, in her journey inwards, she comes across her secret soul, and as an aftermath of this discovery of her own soul, she sees the Divine Mother, the Divine Power which forms and governs the world, descending into her body. Thus says Sri Aurobindo:

A living image of the original Power,
A face, a form came down into her heart
And made of it its temple and pure abode.
But when its feet had touched the quivering bloom,
A mighty movement rocked the inner space
As if a world were shaken and found its soul:
Out of the Inconscient's soulless mindless Night
A flaming serpent rose released from sleep.
It rose billowing its coils and stood erect
And climbing mightily stormily on its way
It touched her centres with its flaming mouth:
As if a fiery kiss had broken their sleep,
They bloomed and laughed surcharged with light and bliss;
Then at the crown it joined the Eternal's space.
In the flower of the head, in the flower of Matter's base,
In each divine stronghold and Nature-knot
It held together the mystic stream which joins
The viewless summits with the unseen depths,
The string of forts that make the frail defence
Safeguarding us against the enormous world,
Our lines of self-expression in its vast.
. . . Powers and divinities burst flaming forth;
Each part of the being trembling with delight
Lay overwhelmed with tides of happiness
And saw her hand in every circumstance
And felt her touch in every limb and cell:
In the country of the lotus of the head
Which thinking mind has made its busy space,
In the castle of the lotus twixt the brows
Whence it shoots the arrows of its sight and will,
In the passage of the lotus of the throat
Where speech must rise and the expressing mind
And the heart's impulse run towards word and fact,

A glad uplift and a new working came. . . .
In the kingdom of the lotus of the heart
Love chanting its pure hymeneal hymn
Made life and body mirrors of sacred joy
And all the emotions gave themselves to God.
In the navel lotus's broad imperial range
Its proud ambitions and its master lusts
Were tamed into instruments of a great calm sway
To do a work of God on earthly soil.
In the narrow nether centre's petty parts
Its childish game of daily dwarf desires
Was changed into a sweet and boisterous play,
A romp of little gods with life in Time.
In the deep place where once the Serpent slept,
There came a grip on Matter's giant powers
For large utilities in life's little space;
A firm ground was made for heaven's descending
    might.
Behind all reigned her sovereign deathless soul . . .

This is a vivid description of the opening of the lotuses in the human system, and the results that ensue in the workings of the mind, life and body with their opening.

We have observed that pranayama, the science of breath, and mantra, the science of the word, are conjoined to effect the awakening of the Kundalini. Necessarily, before the normal human consciousness can rise with this power and merge itself with the super-conscient, there has to be concentration — a concentration of the mind.

There are many methods of concentration. One is to take a form, a word or an idea representing the aspect of the divine which appeals to you and dwell upon it uninterruptedly. There will be the distraction of thoughts, and there are two ways of dealing with them. One is to separate yourself and let the thoughts pass without identifying yourself with them, without sanctioning them, but just watching them. Bereft of this sanction, the thought mind runs down and the speed of the thoughts slowly lessens. Another and a more strenuous method is to exercise your will and keep out every thought the moment it touches the periphery of your mind. Either way the aim is to concentrate the mind on growing towards the superconscient.

Rajayoga recognises that no one can do these mystic operations without a preliminary preparation. That is why this eight-limbed yoga — as it is systematised — speaks of the first two five-limbed disciplines. They are to prepare the moral and the mental being with the necessary purification. They consist, first, of five restraints: not to harm anybody — not only in the physical sense, but also in the mental and the emotional sense. So thoughts that hurt and emotions like hatred, jealousy, anger, must be completely controlled; to abstain from untruth — to think the truth, to act the truth, and to speak the truth; then comes non-stealing — not only not to steal physically what belongs to another, but also not even mentally to appropriate what doesn't really belong to you; next celibacy — the preservation and the upliftment of the sex energy; and lastly non-greediness, not to allow greed to develop in oneself at any level.

Following this discipline of the five restraints are the five observances: purity — this purity, you will understand, is not so much physical as psychological; contentment — not pleasure, but a deep contentment with what God has endowed you; austerity — the massing of the inner forces and the focussing of them on the object, a galvanising of all your energies towards your aim; study — study of the scriptures, mystical literature, experience and realisations of those who have gone before you, literature written by your teacher or other teachers so far as it can help you to widen your horizon; worship and adoration of God — worship not necessarily with external ritual, but the inner adoration of the soul.

Adoration is a vast subject which will form the theme of our talks hereafter.

We are speaking of the eight limbs of this yoga — first the five restraints, then the five observances; then comes posture, asana, which is the putting of the body in such a posture as will enable it to sit immobile, without restlessness for whatever amount of time you expect it to sit. Next comes withdrawal of the mind from the thousand external pre-occupations in which it is spread out normally. After withdrawal comes fixing of the mind on one particular object — not necessarily physical, maybe subtle — and once the mental energies are focussed and fixed, the absorption of the mind on the object — maybe on a form of God, or an idea of God or on the word of God — OM. Once the mind is absorbed, one obtains a certain identity and is completely absorbed in it and lost to all outer awareness. This is what is called samadhi, trance, which is a capital step for a complete merger of your consciousness with the divine consciousness.

The aim of Rajayoga is not merely to attain samadhi, but it also concerns itself with the various mystic powers that are attainable or are effortlessly attained in the course of this yoga. For, as you know, each level of consciousness, each level of being has its characteristic modes of functioning. As higher and higher levels of consciousness are opened up above the physical mind, above the material life, new powers come into operation. Whether one consciously evokes these powers and exercises them — powers such as the capacity of lightening the body, of making it heavy, the power of being in many places at the same time, of seeing ahead, there are eight or nine powers which are called accomplishments — or whether they manifest by themselves, the true yogi does not make much of them. It is only showmen, pseudos, who display these powers, under whatever plea, and try to establish themselves on a superior pedestal. A true seeker, when he becomes aware of these powers, uses them only when he is moved by the inner or the higher will.

Sri Aurobindo concludes this section by saying that while the broad aims of Hathayoga and Rajayoga have, necessarily, got to be included in the comprehensive aim of the Integral Yoga, their laborious physical and psycho-physical methods need not be adopted, though in the preliminary stages they may be made use of. Some, if they find them useful, may continue to use them, but they can only prepare the seeker for the greater glories of the Spirit that are opened by the Integral Yoga.

We have today completed the second part of the *Synthesis of Yoga*, the Yoga of Knowledge. It has taken us nearly a year, and it has been an arduous task to follow Sri Aurobindo in his tracing of the line of development of the Yoga of Knowledge. Now we will have, from the next session onwards, a lighter, more vivid, more appealing task of studying his development of the Yoga of Love. For whoever has come here, whoever has lived under the aegis of the Mother, cannot but breathe the vibrations of Divine Love.

How the seeker awakes to the divinity of love, to the power of creative love, how human love transforms itself into Divine Love, and how love has got its own steps and gradations for the ascent of the human spirit to the highest altitudes of the Divine, all these are narrated in the next seven chapters of the Way of Love.

Questions

I was reading S.'s chronicle for All India Radio on Sri Aurobindo's centenary, where he quotes Sri Aurobindo as saying that when the new creation is about to emerge, all the worst comes up. Could you comment on that?

It is true. Sri Aurobindo has always emphasised that when one undertakes to do yoga, which means a change of human nature, elevation of nature and, ultimately, even the transformation of nature, all that is to be transformed has to come up. There is an intention in nature that the worst has to be pushed to the surface because it is that which has to be transformed. The challenge is posed so that the spirit or the power that is at work may face it, and not shirk from it. Even if it were not a question of the supramental transformation, but a question of the transformation of the ordinary nature, all the difficulties in that nature precipitate themselves to the surface and call for resolution. That is why, the occultists have always said, that before the outbreak of light, before the dawn, there is the darkest night. As our creation has emerged from the inconscient, from the night of the inconscience, there are many knots of that darkness, of that nescience, which have to be resolved. Unless that is done no further progress is possible, no steps can be taken onwards. That is why nature pushes all the hidden difficulties to the surface, in order that they may first be dealt with and progress made really possible. Unless this is done, the progress made is very flimsy and at the first uprush of the neglected difficulties and obscurities it will be held up.

Both Sri Aurobindo and the Mother had always welcomed this exposure of the obscurities in the dark corners of the being when the yogic effort was made in earnest by any individual. They showed great understanding, sympathy and counselled patience before this preliminary clearing was effected.

OTHER IMPORTANT NEW AGE BOOKS

THE YOGA OF LOVE (Based on Sri Aurobindo's Synthesis of Yoga)
—M.P. Pandit

Love is the crown of knowledge. True knowledge ends in love, even as real, wide, spontaneous love which is either vouchsafed to one or springs from the fount of the heart leads one to the perception of the existence of God everywhere. Love opens many windows on the Reality that is God; one cannot escape perceiving God when one is filled with love for God. Even as knowledge culminates in love, love leads to an integral knowledge.

ISBN: 81-7822-057-1

THE YOGA OF SELF-PERFECTION (Based on Sri Aurobindo's Synthesis of Yoga)—*M.P. Pandit*

The Yoga of Self-Perfection recognizes a Divine purpose in life and starts from the premise that the ultimate aim of life is not simply escape, but rather, to work out the divine perfection in manifestation.

ISBN: 81-7822-077-6

THE YOGA OF WORKS (Based on Sri Aurobindo's Synthesis of Yoga)
—M.P. Pandit

The Yoga of Works is perhaps the first and most important aspect of yoga for seekers to take up. It deals with the problems of—energy, action and direction which confronts us all whenever we try to integrate our spiritual aspirations with the daily life around us and the need to "work" in the society and play a role in the vast undertakings of the Western world.

ISBN: 81-7822-079-2

KUNDALINI YOGA (A Brief Study of Sir John Woodroff's "The Serpent Power")—*M.P. Pandit*

The search for inner awakening and unfolding of hidden powers has brought man to the threshold of the last frontier: himself. For it is deep within that we find the secret key and unlock the door long held secure from our sight. The ancient philosopher's call "Know Thyself" continues to beckon us on the path of knowledge as the final object of our ongoing investigation.

ISBN: 81-7822-076-8

THE BOOK OF CHAKRA HEALING—*Liz Simpson*

The Book of Chakra Healing is a comprehensive guide to the ancient Indian system of chakras. These centres of "spinning energy" in the body help to maintain your physical, mental, emotional, and spiritual balance. This book offers practical way to work on your chakras and shows you how to unblock and rebalance your energy. This book will be of great benefit to both health care professionals and lay people and will inspire many to explore and develop their relationship with an integral part of their being—the chakras.

ISBN: 81-7822-043-1

THE SELF-REVEALED KNOWLEDGE THAT LIBERATES THE SPIRIT —*Roy Eugene Davis*

In this book the author presents a clear explanation of the soul's awakening through progressive stages of spiritual growth from ordinary, illusional states of awareness to mental illumination, spiritual enlightenment, and liberation of consciousness. The descriptions of philosophical principles will satisfy the rational mind and speak to the heart that aspires to direct perception of truth.

ISBN: 81-7822-050-4

THE HEALING HANDBOOK (A Spiritual Guide to Healing Yourself and Others)—*Tara Ward*

In this book the author presents a range of techniques and tools for healing yourself and other, including children and animals. The book features: Techniques for chakra awareness, relaxation, self-assessment, releasing anger and resentment, healing physical conditions, creating a healing sanctuary, increasing sensitivity, developing intuition, protecting yourself, absent healing and provides information about healing tools such as pendulums, crystals, colour, sound, massage, spirit guides.

ISBN: 81-7822-034-2

HEALING THE FUTURE (The Journey Within)—*Deepak Kashyap*

The greatest possibilities of body-cure, says the author, lie in forgetting the body. To the extent we lose body-consciousness and identify with the Spirit, physical disability and mental trauma disappearing on their own. *Healing the Future* is then, an attempted tip-off on the little secrets of holistic living that can be mastered in easy, small steps. This book urges you to treat consciousness as a canvas, and begin adding new colour, shine and texture to your tomorrow from this very instant.

ISBN: 81-7822-039-3

STRESS-FREE WORK WITH YOGA AND AYURVEDA —*Vinod Verma*

Dr. Verma's advice for a stress-free work environment begins with a daily yoga program. The aim of this book is to provide a guide for building a better work atmosphere based on an understanding of Ayurvedic personality types—according to your fundamental nature or *prakriti*. It is also important to learn how to acquire a state of satisfaction in your personal life, which is essential for both better work performance and your health. It helps you to build your own good atmosphere—even in the worst of circumstances.

ISBN: 81-7822-000-8

CHAKRA ENERGY MASSAGE (Spiritual Evolution into the Subconscious Through Activation of the Energy Points of the Feet)—*Marianne Uhl*

This book guides you into the fascinating world of the energy body. Drawing on the knowledge gained by Foot Reflexology Massage, it introduces you to the Chakra Energy Massage. By means of the fine energy channels connecting them to the body's organs and energy centres, our feet reflect our physical and psychic condition. It enables you to acquire basic knowledge needed for Foot Reflexology Massage and Chakra Energy Massage.

ISBN: 81-7822-004-0

THE SPIRITUAL BASIS OF REAL PROSPERITY —*Roy Eugene Davis*

In this book the author proclaims that life need not be difficult, painful, or limited. He clearly explains how anyone who is capable of rational thinking can be spiritually awake and serenely happy, live creatively and effectively, have life-enhancing desires easily fulfilled, and consistently accomplish meaningful purposes.

ISBN: 81-7822-053-9

ART AS A GUIDE TO SELF-REALIZATION—*J. Donald Walters*

Art as a Guide to Self-Realization offers a blueprint for the future of art, and shows how art can be a powerful influence for meaningful existence and positive attitudes in society. The book presents a new approach to the arts, one that views both artistic expression and artistic appreciation as creative communication.

ISBN: 81-7822-028-8

SUPERCONSCIOUSNESS (**How to Benefit from Emerging Spiritual Trends**) —*J. Donald Walters*

The book explains the emerging techniques and attitudes that will help ease the transition to a more spiritually nurturing society and teaches us to awaken the seeds of intuition, freedom, and joy that lies dormant within each of us. This is the first book that applies the teachings of the great sage Paramhansa Yogananda (1893-1952, author of *Autobiography of a Yogi*) to the 21st Century.

ISBN: 81-7822-026-1

THE INTUITIVE WAY (**A Guide To Living From Inner Wisdom**)—*Penney Peirce*

It demonstrates practical applications from speeding decision making to expanding personal growth and makes you aware about the following benefits of active intuition:• A positive, life-enhancing attitude • More synchronicity and good luck • Greater efficiency with less effort • Attention to detail while seeing the big picture • Increased creativity and imagination • Confidence in your own insights • Understanding your soul's purpose.

ISBN: 81-7822-008-3

PSYCHIC POWERS **A Practical Guide Awaken Your Sixth Sense**—*Melita Denning Osborne Phillips*

This practical guide offers complete step-by-step instructions on developing your innate psychic skills in divination, dowsing, clairvoyance, psychometry, and spirit communication. You will learn how to safely enhance your mental and psychic abilities, and to use your abilities to positively change your life and the lives of those around you.

ISBN: 81-7822-051-2

SPIRITUAL HEALING (**Doctors Examine Therapeutic Touch and other Holistic treatments**)—*Dora Kunz*

Healing is a divine art. The book presents a surprising open-mindedness and forward looking vision. A spiritual revolution is underway in health care. More and more doctors, nurses, and counselors are recognizing that health means treating the soul and the psyche as well as the body.

ISBN: 81-7822-011-3